201

SECRETS of a

HIGH-PERFORMANCE
DENTAL PRACTICE

201 SECRETS of a
HIGH-PERFORMANCE DENTAL PRACTICE

BOB LEVOY

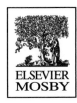

ELSEVIER
MOSBY

ELSEVIER
MOSBY

11830 Westline Industrial Drive
St. Louis, Missouri 63146

ISBN-13: 978-0-323-02869-1
ISBN-10: 0-323-02869-1

Publishing Director: Linda Duncan
Executive Editor: Penny Rudolph
Associate Developmental Editor: Courtney Sprehe
Publishing Services Manager: Pat Joiner
Project Manager: Rachel E. Dowell
Design Project Manager: Bill Drone

Printed in the United States of America

Last digit is the print number: 9 8 7 6

For Martha . . . again.
More than ever.

About the Author

As president of Success Dynamics Inc., Bob Levoy has conducted over 3000 seminars for a wide range of business and professional groups throughout North America and overseas. Among them have been hundreds of dental associations, academies, local societies, and schools of dentistry.

His unique background in industry and the healthcare professions has focused on market research and the development of programs to improve the performance and profitability of professional practices.

Bob holds three college degrees in business and professional fields. He has written five previous books and hundreds of articles on management topics. Currently, he is a monthly columnist and Editorial Board member for numerous publications in the healthcare professions.

For information about his availability as a speaker for your organization, contact Success Dynamics Inc. (516) 626-1353 or b.levoy@att.net.

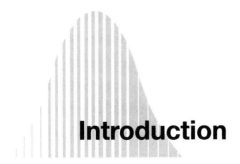

Introduction

There are many definitions of high performance. The Malcolm Baldridge National Quality Award Program created by Congress defines it as, "Work approaches used to systematically pursue ever higher levels of overall organizational and individual performance, including quality, productivity, innovation rate, and cycle time performance."*

The term *high-performance dental practice* used in this book refers to *above-average levels of:*

case acceptance
patient loyalty
patient referrals
patient satisfaction
practice growth
productivity
profitability
referrals from colleagues, physicians, etc.
staff retention
teamwork

Above-average achievement in these categories places high-performance dental practices at the upper end (shaded portion) of the familiar *bell-shaped curve* shown throughout this book. This curve, the most widely used model in statistics, depicts a frequency distribution with the percent of dental practices shown on the vertical

---

*Baldridge National Quality Program 2004, Criteria for Performance Excellence.

ordinate (from low to high) and the magnitude of each achievement depicted on the horizontal ordinate (from below average on the left to above average on the right).

What does this select group of high-performance dental practices have in common to have attained these above-average achievements? The answer in simplest terms: *they have the right people, in the right jobs, doing the right things, at the right time.*

Obviously, there's more to the story—all of which will unfold in this book.

Real practices. Real solutions.

In the course of my career, I've had the privilege of conducting over 3000 seminars for a wide range of business and professional groups throughout North America and overseas. As part of the market research for these programs, I continue to visit countless professional practices not only in dentistry, but also in medicine, podiatry, optometry, physical therapy, veterinary medicine, accounting, and law, among others. It has enabled me to meet hundreds of high-performance practitioners in each of these professions and ask them such questions as:

- What makes your practice so successful?
- What are you doing differently than others to account for your success?
- What are the secrets of hiring top-notch employees and how do you keep them motivated?
- What have been your toughest management problems and how did you solve them?
- What do you wish you had done differently?
- What lessons did you learn that may help others avoid costly mistakes?

The answers to these questions became the framework of this book.

Let's begin.

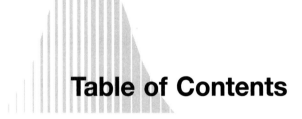

Table of Contents

Chapter 3: Take Your Practice to the Next Level: Make It a "Brand"   44

Chapter 4: Long-Range Strategic Planning   63

Chapter 5: Golden Opportunities for Practice Growth 69

Chapter 6: Secrets of Savvy Networking 81

Chapter 7: Patient Expectations, Satisfaction, and Loyalty 100

Chapter 8: Secrets of Successful Case Presentations 119

Chapter 13: Secrets of Staff Retention — 207

Chapter 14: Build a High-Performance Team — 221

Chapter 15: Action Steps to Ignite Practice Growth — 237

201

SECRETS of a

HIGH-PERFORMANCE
DENTAL PRACTICE

1

Be Different. Or Better. Preferably Both.

At a recent seminar, business guru Tom Peters said that private practice owners must create something special to stand out in a world of surpluses. He noted that we live in a surplus society: a society full of similar companies employing people with similar educational backgrounds and experiences who have similar ideas, producing similar things that have similar quality and similar prices.[1]

He was talking to physical therapists. But his description of a surplus, commoditized society is equally true for dentists. The solution in both cases is *differentiation*.

1 Avoid the "commodity trap"

A *commodity* is a product that is perceived to be more or less identical to other similiar products in the same category. Sugar, nails, and cotton are examples. Typically, the only determinant of a commodity's value is price. Quality is assumed to be identical unless consumers hear otherwise.

Unfortunately many patients also think of dentistry as a "commodity" that is standard in all respects, regardless of who does it. To their way of thinking, a crown is a crown and a cleaning is a cleaning, so why not have dental procedures done as inexpensively as possible?

This lack of differentiation causes a vicious cycle. Patients are influenced by "cost" because they don't perceive a difference between one dental practice and another. Dentists, on the other hand, believing that such patients are strictly cost-driven, fail to address the commodity image of their practices and fail to do what's needed to give them a competitive advantage. So the problem persists.

The best way, in fact the *only* way, to avoid the commodity trap is to *differentiate* your practice. Make it unique. Have something about your practice that sets it apart from others in what professor Michael Porter of Harvard University calls "substantial and sustainable ways." That's what will give your practice a *competitive advantage*. Position it at the high end of the bell-shaped curve. And make it *impervious* to competition and "price comparisons."

REALITY CHECK

If what you're doing in your practice is no better, no different (or *perceived* to be no better or different) than what's being done in offices that charge less, then what incentive do patients have to be in your practice? As William James observed, "A difference that makes no difference is not a difference."

The following are among the many, varied ways that high-performance dentists have differentiated their practices. Think of them as a menu of possibilities.

2 Determine your primary focus

Two very different and very important dimensions exist in organizational performance: organizational *efficiency* and organizational *effectiveness*. In deciding how to differentiate your practice, it's important to decide whether your primary focus is going to be on achieving a more *efficient* practice or a more *effective* one.

An efficient practice focuses on *doing things in the right way* to maximize productivity and profitability. An effective practice, on the other hand, focuses on *doing the right things* that maximize patient satisfaction and referrals. The first is an "inward" view. The latter is an "outward" view.

Dentists who are focused on efficiency often look for ways to maximize profitability by working faster, delegating as much as possible, skimping on payroll expenses, and cutting corners to save time or money. And these are sound management strategies, up to a point. Being efficient definitely has survival value in the highly competitive, cost-conscious economy of managed care.

The point of diminishing returns occurs when such cost-containment measures impinge on patient satisfaction. For example, does the emphasis on delegation and working faster require a dentist to take less time with patients to learn their needs, properly explain findings and recommendations, and answer questions? Does skimping on payroll expenses result in a practice being understaffed at times or, worse, having a staff that is not as knowledgeable and experienced as the job requires? Does belt-tightening require a cutback on continuing education or state-of-the-art equipment? Alas, you can be efficient without being effective.

REALITY CHECK

Thomas J. Neff and James C. Citrin, chairman and managing director, respectively, of Spencer Stuart, an executive search firm, offer the following definition of success. "Contrary to conventional wisdom, business success is not just defined by revenue and profit growth, superior return on equity or increased shareholder value. Rather, in our view, business success is doing the right things. When chief executives succeed in doing the right things with their companies and their businesses, the traditional measures of performance inevitably follow."[2]

FROM THE SUCCESS FILES

"For several years Scott Coleman, DDS, Houston, TX, viewed his practice as an 'insurance driven machine.' Working with several patients each day, he eventually expanded his staff to 16 members. But even though his practice was booming, Dr. Coleman was dissatisfied. 'I'm not a big fan of roaming from chair to chair, trying to see four patients at a time,' he explains. 'My patients didn't receive my full attention, and I couldn't provide the full level of service they deserved.'"

To get his practice to a manageable level and offer patients a more pleasant atmosphere, Dr. Coleman selectively reviewed his existing patients, shifted the practice's focus to cosmetic dentistry, and reduced his staff. "The practice is making more money," he says, "but more importantly, I feel better knowing that I can spend a significant amount of time with each patient and do my level best to meet their desires with regard to oral health."[3]

HARD-LEARNED LESSON
Management expert Peter Drucker said it best: "Nothing is less productive than to make more efficient what should not be done at all."[4]

---

3 Commit to excellence

"There is considerable evidence," William Andres, former chairman of the Dayton-Hudson Corporation, told the Harvard Business School Marketing Club, "that the very best businesses concentrate almost single-mindedly, on serving the customer. Pleasing customers," he said, "is an *obsession*. Service is an *obsession*. Quality is an *obsession*. Dependability is an *obsession*. Attention to detail is an *obsession*."

His advice is dead-on for any service-driven business, dentistry included.

The word *obsession* is the key. It implies not just a "lip service" promise to do these things, but rather a no excuses, unswerving *commitment* to quality, service, dependability, and attention to detail.

For many practices, *growth* is king. For high-performance dental practices, *excellence* is king.

FROM THE SUCCESS FILES
"Become a "Quality Specialist" and create an office that exudes that image," says William G. Dickerson, DDS, FAACD, Las Vegas, NV. "My net income tripled in the first year I adopted this philosophy."[5]

"One thing is almost a certainty," says Peter E. Dawson, DDS, St. Petersburg, FL, founder and director of the Dawson Center for Advanced Dental Study. "The day you make the decision to have a truly superior practice based on clinical excellence, your enjoyment of dentistry will go up. It will be a decision that only can be beneficial for both you and your patients."[6]

"The best advice I can give anyone is to focus on practice excellence from day one," says Edward Lowe, DMD, Vancouver, British Columbia, Canada. "Be the best you can be and do everything as well as you can. Never compromise your education."[7]

HARD-LEARNED LESSONS

"The truth is, as with any business venture, an unshakable foundation of quality and service is what drives success," says K. William Mopper, DDS, MS, Winnetka, IL. "If you demonstrate that you can consistently deliver excellent esthetics, produce functional restorations that last and charge fair fees, this area of your practice will grow naturally and exponentially."[8]

"First be *best*, then be *first*." These words, spoken by Grant Tinker when he became chairman of NBC, articulate the philosophy that guided the network to its number one position during his tenure.

In today's highly competitive environment, good enough is simply not good enough.

4 Magnification

"Most dentists who use loupes," says the *CRA Newsletter* published by Clinical Research Associates, "state with conviction that magnification not only increases the quality of their treatment, it also increases their speed because they can see what they are doing better."[9]

FROM THE SUCCESS FILES

"You cannot provide excellence in cosmetic dentistry without some form of enhanced vision," says Michael Sesemann, DDS, Omaha, NE. "Loupes take you to a whole new level, allowing you to see as well as feel when working. All members of my staff use loupes."[10]

"The next step in enhanced visualization," says Arturo Garcia, DDS, Wayne, PA, "is a dental microscope."[11]

"The microscope has raised the bar of excellence for restorative dentistry," say Cherilyn G. Sheets, DDS, and prosthodontist Jacinthe M. Paquette, DDS, Newport Beach, CA. "The ultimate marginal fit of restorations can be enhanced due to more refined preparations, improved impression accuracy, and better assessment of marginal fit during the try-in and final luting. The highest-quality dental laboratories use microscopes for a broad spectrum of dental laboratory bench procedures. Having clinical magnification equal to laboratory magnification improves the jointly produced final product and greatly reduces the need for laboratory requested re-preparations or impressions. The ultimate winner is the patient who receives restorative care with idealized tissue response, aesthetics, and longevity."[12]

"When dentists make the commitment to enhance their vision," Dr. Garcia says, "they are making a commitment to excellence, both in their skills and in patient communication."[11]

5 A thorough oral cancer exam

"Oral and pharyngeal cancers are diagnosed in about 30,000 Americans annually," reports the surgeon general in Oral Health in America. "8000 die from these diseases each year. These cancers are primarily diagnosed in the elderly. Prognosis is poor. The 5 year survival rate for white patients is 56 percent; for blacks, it is only 34 percent."[13]

"One national survey," it continues, referring to a 1995 report, "found that only 14 percent of adults 40 and older reported that they ever had an oral cancer examination. Of these only 7 percent had an exam within the last year."

ACTION STEP
"Do a thorough oral examination on every patient every six months to a year," says Myer Leonard, DDS, Golden Valley, MN. "This exam should go beyond recording the cavities and restorations, pocket depths, and missing teeth. You should conscientiously inspect the tongue, the palate, the floor of the mouth, the buccal mucosa, the fauces, etc. This means determining whether all the tissues are normal and healthy."

And be sure, he adds, to tell your patients what you are doing and why you are doing it.[14]

Countless dentists and hygienists have told me that after such examinations, patients often say, "That's the most thorough exam I've ever had" or "You're the first dentist (or hygienist) to do such an exam."

THE NEXT STEP

"In the past," says Scott Benjamin DDS, Sidney, NY, "I often encountered patients with suspicious lesions who simply didn't take this concern very seriously. All of this changed," he adds, "since I started using digital photography. Today, any time we see an oral lesion, we photo-document it. When patients realize a lesion is important enough to photograph, they take it more seriously. This has had an enormous impact on my patients' acceptance of my treatment recommendations."[15]

 State-of-the-art equipment

"From the patient's point of view," says Charles D. Samaras, DMD, Lowell, MA, "up-to-date dental technology provides for better patient care and service through patient education, thorough diagnosis, increased communication, and greater efficiency. Patients accept the premise that "high tech" usually connotes high quality because patients have become consumers. The higher quality treatment and service that technology provides is a competitive necessity, not only to maintain your patient base but also to attract new patients to your practice—new patients that desire quality treatment and service and are willing to pay for it. In addition, the technology will enable you present more thorough, more comprehensive case presentations with a corresponding increase in case acceptance."[16]

FROM THE SUCCESS FILES

"Let me summarize some of the many benefits of digital radiography," says Jeffrey B. Dalin, DDS, FACD, FAGD, FICD, St. Louis, MO. "Less radiation exposure to patients, instant on-screen images, rapid and superior diagnoses, image-enhancement capabilities (such as magnification, contrast, and coloring), improved patient acceptance and education, total elimination of the darkroom, chemicals, and film, and easy image-sharing with other dentists or third party payers."[17]

"In my personal experience," says Stewart Rosenberg, DDS, Laurel, MD, "I know of no better return on investment for our practice than our purchase of a YSGG hard and soft tissue laser . . . It's a tremendous practice builder to offer needle-free, drill-free dentistry. These factors have a positive economic impact on our practices and are enough to more than justify the cost of the laser."

"However," Dr. Rosenberg adds, "the real economic and professional bonanza is the array of procedures we can now offer our patients that we used to either refer to specialists, or worse, ignore completely. These procedures represent a gold mine of incremental income walking in and out of our doors on a daily basis. And best of all, we're doing our patients a great service by addressing their needs more comprehensively, more comfortably, and often more economically—and have a lot of fun in the process."[18]

"When asked what contributes to increased revenue as a result of using a laser, more than half of respondents in surveys by *Dental Products Report* "indicated additional procedures, better patient acceptance and retention, and increased productivity. Almost half reported gaining new patients and about one-third increased their fees and began performing higher-end procedures."[19]

HARD-LEARNED LESSON

"Patients repeatedly state that when practices utilize advanced technology in the delivery of care," says Eugene L. Antenucci, DDS, FAGD, Huntington, NY, "they perceive they are actually receiving better care. Patients' perceptions of enhanced quality of care create greater degrees of trust in the ability of the office to treat them in the manner they want to be treated. Whether we like it or not, patients tend to equate advanced technology with better care, perceiving that the doctors and staff are more "up-to-date" and are more concerned with the patient's comfort and well-being."[20]

REALITY CHECK

The question isn't "How can I afford this new technology?" says Glenn A. MacFarlane, DMD, founding member and past president of the New Jersey Academy of Cosmetic Dentistry, but rather, "How can I afford *not* to have this new technology?"[21]

7 An informative, user-friendly Web site

"An effective Web site is no longer a convenient option," reports the *Blair/McGill Advisory,* "but a practical necessity for doctors seeking to maximize their practice's growth potential. A comprehensive well-designed Web site can give your practice a competitive advantage."[22]

Commonly found features include the following:

History and philosophy of the practice
Services provided
Fax/phone numbers and office hours
Photos of the office
Directions to the office including a map
Photos and short biographies of the dentist(s) and staff members
Articles on various dental health topics with links to related Web sites
Current and past issues of practice newsletters
Answers to frequently asked questions
Before and after photographs of aesthetic treatment
Online appointment scheduling
An e-mail link
Downloadable forms such as a new patient registration form or medical/dental history form that can be filled out at home and forwarded electronically to the office. This feature saves time for patients (while at the office) and for the staff.

"The fact is the Internet provides practices a wealth of opportunities to enhance patient relationships, none more powerful or valuable than in the area of communications," say Caludio Levato, DDS, Bloomingdale, IL, and Barry Feydberg, DDS, Skokie, IL. "Many options exist to help you improve communication with your peers, your laboratory and your patients."[23]

FROM THE SUCCESS FILES
"Patients in Hendersonville, TN can make a dental appointment with George A. Bare, DMD, with a click of the mouse," says technology expert Cheryl Farr. "Or they can call the practice. The important thing is that they get a choice, providing them with a higher level of service than they will get from many practices."[24]

REALITY CHECK

A study by Arthur Anderson showed that more than 83% of Internet users are likely to leave a Web site if they feel they have to make too many clicks to find what they're looking for.[25] Among other Web site problems: confusing navigation, slow page loads, long scrolling pages.

ACTION STEP

"There are many ways to create an office Web site," says Gary Osias, OD, San Lorenzo, CA, "but I only recommend one. Seek out the help of a professional designer and pay to have a Web site that impresses Internet surfers. Homegrown Web sites appear obviously amateur to professional computer users, and when professional computer users search the Web, they base their first impression of a business by the quality of its Web site."[26]

HARD-LEARNED LESSON

"With the right content on your site and a strong e-mail communication system," says DentistryOnline.Inc, "you re-enfranchise yourself with your patient base, become their source for information about dentistry, create greater patient loyalty, and increase referrals. In fact, your Web site can become one of your strongest internal marketing tools."[27]

---

8 An in-office lab

The following quote is from the Web site of Charles J. Miller DDS, S. Rand Werrin, DDS, and John W. Gruendel, DMD, Pittsburgh, PA.

"Our unique in-house dental laboratory provides the very finest in dental technology and artistry. As one of the only in-house dental labs in Pittsburgh, we can offer our patients a full range of services as well as faster service and the highest quality products."

"We are able to meticulously supervise the progress of your case as it flows through the laboratory process. We have complete control over the techniques, the material and the quality. The combination of leading edge technology and very talented technicians assures that the service we extend to you is the finest quality available."

In addition, this page has photographs of each of their four dental laboratory technicians at their workstations and an explanation of each of their respective roles in the fabrication process.

On the information page of the Web site, and as part of their policy on emergencies, the following information is included: "Since we have our own in-house dental laboratory, our response time to your dental accident can be much shorter than using a dental office that is limited to a commercial or mail-order dental laboratory."[28]

9 Paperless dentistry

"Paperless dentistry," says Linh Bauer, DDS, San Jose, CA, "is more than just moving your hardcopy files to a computer. It's about being able to access patient information *anywhere in your office at any time.* It's about taking anything you would find in a patient file and making it available to those who need it when they need it."

"Patients notice the difference between paperless offices and other offices," Dr. Bauer says. "The ability to store literally everything within the software provides a clean, clutter-free atmosphere. Void of file cabinets, the office shows our patients that we are well organized and advanced. The moment a patient enters our practice, I am confident everything I need for that visit—X-rays, medical history, etc.—is legible, clear and will be found in the patient's file."[29]

REALITY CHECK

"To look at digital records and wonder if that's a return on investment in the dollar sense, the answer is absolutely," says Barry K. Freydberg, DDS, Skokie, IL. He cites the amount of staff hours spent searching for records, or worse yet, losing a record. Dr. Freydberg also notes the time taken to write letters to patients or specialists. 'Digital records aren't just a game or a toy anymore, they're truly a cost-savings."[30]

HARD-LEARNED LESSON

"A simple equation sums it up," Dr. Bauer says. "Paperless = Clutterless = Less Stress = Improved Quality of Life = A Happy Dentist."[29]

10 An office free of "architectural barriers"

The Americans with Disabilities Act requires businesses to be accessible to the disabled. Yet many dental offices have distant parking; stairs; protruding thresholds or narrow entranceways that place restrictions on the accessibility of their offices for the 43 million Americans—more than one out of seven—who are physically disabled.

Compliance with ADA guidelines makes your practice more accessible to individuals with wheelchairs or other supportive devices. And the numbers are increasing as more people are living longer and in many cases becoming mobility-impaired.

Dentists and staff who understand and accommodate the needs of this sizable group will earn the good will and referrals of these patients, as well as those of their families and friends.

FROM THE SUCCESS FILES

A newsletter from the office of Albert Ousborne, DDS, Thomas Keller, DDS, and Patrick Ousborne, DDS, Towson, MD, states: "As many of our patients have the need for a wheelchair, we can now provide one during your visit to our office. We felt this would be helpful so that our patients would not need to bring their own or may find one helpful in coming from the parking lot to their appointment. Just ask. We are always seeking ways to better serve you."[31]

11 An attractive, up-to-date office

What kind of image does your office convey, and is it congruent with the level of professionalism you want to project and the quality of care you provide? The fact is, you don't have a choice as to whether your office makes a statement or not. The only choice is what kind of statement.

FROM THE SUCCESS FILES

"If you are contemplating remodeling, or building a new facility," says orthodontist Richard J. Resler, DDS, Saginaw, MI, "I would strongly urge you to 'go for it.' At age 53, debt free and working in an office that was very adequate and profitable, I made the decision that I wanted to spend the rest of my working career in a state-of-the-art facility that would afford me all of the modern comforts and advantages. Consequently, 14 months and $700,000 later, I have achieved that goal."

"The results," says Dr. Resler, "have been remarkable. While production increased 12 percent immediately, we are operating with much reduced stress and a very much-improved doctor and staff attitude. Patients have made our office the talk of the town, and new exams have increased without additional promotion. As a result, I can see the extra expense will easily be covered in a few years."[32]

HARD-LEARNED LESSON

One of the most often-heard regrets from dentists is the following: "I didn't remodel (or redecorate) my office sooner." In many cases, dentists add, "I never realized how bad it was until we redecorated and everyone told us how nice it was and what a big improvement it was."

Every 7 years, you need to either redecorate or move. Even if you don't notice the sameness, your patients will.

The following sign seen in an interior decorator's office offers wisdom for the new dentist: "The longer your office says struggling dentist, the longer the struggle."

12 Available for emergencies

"Patients in pain or in need of an appointment quickly become every practice's best missionaries," says consultant Linda Miles. "They will tell multiple people if they were treated with dignity and respect. They will tell even more people if their cry for help was treated with total disregard or not at all. Turning away those in pain is anti-marketing one's own practice."[33]

REALITY CHECK

Some "emergency patients" are in need of immediate care. Others aren't, and simply use an "emergency" as an excuse to get a same-day appointment. It's also true that some "emergency patients" never return for the balance of their treatment, and others, sad to say, never pay their bills.

ACTION STEPS

Unless the numbers of emergency patients are getting out of hand, consider having your receptionist say the following to such callers:

(To screen them) "Are you hurting so badly that you need to be seen immediately? ("Did it keep you awake at night?")

(To accommodate them) "How soon can you get here?" ("You may have to wait, but the doctor will do something to help you.")

FROM THE SUCCESS FILES

Just as the office of Wayne Pulver, DDS, an endodontist in Toronto, Canada, was ready to close one evening, a patient called to say he was in terrible pain, and asked to see the doctor as soon as possible. The person was desperate. The two endodontists whom he had already called were unable to see him that evening.

Dr. Pulver's receptionist asked, "How soon can you get here?"

"20 to 30 minutes," the patient replied,

"We'll wait for you," she said.

The patient was subsequently seen, appropriately treated, called later that evening by Dr. Pulver and, in the days following, seen for the balance of treatment.

As it turned out, this stranger to the practice was one of the wealthiest, most influential people in Canada, and needless to say, most appreciative of Dr. Pulver's kindness.

"Our position on emergencies," states the Web site of the Atlanta, GA, Center for Cosmetic Dentistry, "is very simple: If you think it is an emergency, then we do too."[34]

13 On-time for appointments

Being "on time" gives your practice a competitive advantage in today's time-pressured environment. It sends a message as well, because in our society time spent waiting is linked to *status*. The more important you are, the more promptly you're seen. VIPs never wait.

Martha Zarnow, a vice president of Viacom International, was quoted in the *Wall Street Journal* on why she fired her obstetrician after an extended stay in his waiting room. "I'm a busy professional. I don't make people wait for me and I don't expect to be kept waiting. Whenever I notice that kind of arrogance, I switch doctors."[35]

REALITY CHECK

How long will patients remain good-natured about waiting beyond their appointment time? 15 minutes, according to a study of 10,000 patients interviewed by National Research Corporation of Lincoln, NE.

HARD-LEARNED LESSONS
- Anxiety makes waiting seem longer.
- Uncertain waits are longer than known, finite waits
- Unexplained waits are longer than explained waits
- Unfair waits are longer than equitable waits

When you do fall behind in schedule, a sincere "I'm sorry you had to wait so long" really does have a mellowing effect on the patient.

FROM THE SUCCESS FILES

Among the items on the Web site of Ian Shuman, DDS, Baltimore, MD, is his "Philosophy of Time." "We know that you have reserved time in your busy life because caring for your dental health is important to you. We value your time and we pride ourselves on running on schedule."

"We also believe in family time, so the practice hours are designed so that evenings are spent with family. We also understand that emergencies do happen and in the event of a dental emergency Dr. Shuman can be reached after hours."[36]

QUESTIONS TO CONSIDER
- Do you have a philosophy of time? Does your staff know it? Has it been put into practice?

HARD-LEARNED LESSON

"If you can stay on time for appointments 90 percent of the time," says Neil Gailmard, OD, MBA, Munster, IN, "you will stand out as a shining example in a sea of mediocrity. Becoming an "on time practice" is good for patient relations, and it reduces stress on your staff."[37]

14 Attention to detail

Author Seth Godin recalls a trainer at American Airlines who always used the following example to explain the critical importance of details: "Every day thousands of employees work incredibly hard to ensure a passenger's loyalty to American Airlines. But if a reservation was wrong, or the ticket was written out incorrectly, or the flight got out late, or the crew wasn't friendly, or the bag was missing, it didn't matter to the passenger that everything else was perfect. One mistake by one employee could mean that the work of thousands, from the corporate office to the maintenance hangars to the cockpit crew, had gone for naught."[38]

HARD-LEARNED LESSON
"Patients will more readily forgive treatment," says Joel Lang, DPM, Cheverly, MD, "than errors in arithmetic. Be diligent about keeping accounts straight. One billing error will irritate most patients—two errors will most assuredly lose a patient."[39]

15 Extended hours

Because of job pressures and time constraints, fewer people than ever are able (or want to) take time off from work for a dental appointment. Extended office hours, whether in the morning or evening, have become if not an imperative, at least an important consideration—especially if other offices have them.

If you're not sure whether your patients would prefer extended hours in the morning or the evening, ask them. Keep it simple, as in the following survey question: "We're considering a change in office hours to serve you better: Would early morning appointments starting at (fill in a time) make coming to our office more convenient for you? (yes)_____(no)_____comments_____"

"Early morning" or "evening appointments" may mean different things to different people. Be sure to specify the exact times you're considering for extended hours, as well as the day(s) of the week. Consider also distributing such a survey only to your "best patients" (i.e., those whom you would like to see more of in your practice). Reason: there's a good chance their preference for office hours will be representative of non-patients like them.

Early morning hours attract what many dentists refer to as "no nonsense" patients, often more concerned with time than money. So, they're in and out and on their way. Many practitioners report these early hour appointments are among the most popular and productive of the day, and are booked far in advance.

FROM THE SUCCESS FILES

"On Thursdays, I start my workday at 6:30 a.m. and end it at 2 p.m.," says Albert L. Ousborne, Jr., DDS, Towson, MD. "This allows our "early-riser patients" an opportunity to come in prior to work. We've had only one opening in the eight years since we started at this hour."[40]

"Schedule new child patients (3 to 5 years old) as well as difficult young operative patients early in the morning," says national speaker Janet Hagerman, RDH. "Children are more cooperative when they are not tired. You too, will be fresher."[41]

16 Language fluency

"Nearly 1 in 5 Americans speaks a language other than English at home, the Census Bureau says, after a surge of nearly 50 percent during the past decade. Most speak Spanish, followed by Chinese, with Russian rising fast."[42]

"Toronto, Canada, once a homogeneous city of staid British tradition, now counts more than 40 percent of the people as foreign born. There are nearly 2000 ethnic restaurants and local radio and television stations broadcast in more than 30 languages."[43]

If like many communities in North America, yours has significant numbers of non-English or limited English–speaking people with whom neither you nor your staff are able to converse, your practice is at a terrible disadvantage—especially if other practices have multi-lingual personnel.

FROM THE SUCCESS FILES

"If you have a large non-English speaking base, you may want to hire multi-lingual staff members," says Neil J. Gajjar, DDS, Mississauga, Ontario, Canada, whose staff speaks five different languages. "Speaking the same language as the patient automatically makes them feel more at home."[44]

ACTION STEPS

- Hire associates and/or staff members fluent in the language of the target populations you would like to attract to your office.
- If you are near a college or university, hire an exchange student for part-time work in your office as an interpreter.
- Offer to pay the tuition for a staff member willing to take an adult education course in the language needed for your practice: 125% of the costs for an "A" in the course, and once the course is completed, give the person a raise.
- *Spanish Terminology for the Dental Team,* published by Elsevier/ Mosby, can be ordered at: www.us.elsevierhealth.com/ product.jsp?isbn=0323025366.
- Another do-it-yourself resource: Audio-Forum offers 285 audiocassette courses in 103 different languages. These vary in length from 1½ hours (key phrases and vocabulary only) to 15 to 20 hours of recorded material. (A catalog of self-instructional language courses is available from: Audio-Forum, One Orchard Park Road, Madison, CT 06443; 800-243-1234; www.audioforum.com.)
- A health history form is available in 21 languages to address today's communication barriers between dentists and their patients. The form uses languages that account for 87.7% of the languages spoken in the United States. MetLife and the University of the Pacific, School of Dentistry, made the Multi-Language Health History Form available at no cost as a PDF file at www.dental.uop.edu under Dental Professionals.[45]

"We know that medical history is an important part of oral health care, but some patients don't have a history on file," says Susan Baker of MetLife Dental. "We also know that doctors don't want to turn away a patient who's in pain, just because of a language barrier. The translations will provide information the dentist can understand and quickly, and it's wonderful for patients to feel that someone has taken the time to do this."[46]

FROM THE SUCCESS FILES

The home page of the Web site for the North Suburban
   Dental Associates in Skokie, IL, has the following announcement:

We Understand! In addition to English, we also have staff members who speak fluent German, Polish, Philippine, Russian, Spanish, Bosnian, Serbian, Croatian, Assyrian, and a "bissel" Yiddish

---

Next to the text are colorful flags to represent each of these cultures.[47]

"Ten years ago, I began practicing in Newport News, VA," says internist Brooks A. Mick, MD, "amid the largest concentration of military posts in the world. Because of service personnel who married overseas and former military people who've tended to settle in this area, there are many folks here whose primary language is Korean, Vietnamese, Japanese, Spanish or Tagalog (Filipino). I try to greet each patient in his or her own language and it has become something of a ritual to ask every patient who speaks a new language to teach me a few words. It's remarkable how much goodwill a single phrase can promote."[48]

17 E.T.D.B.W.

Consultant Michael Hammer in his book, *"The Agenda: What Every Business Must Do To Dominate The Decade"* writes that companies must do a better job of organizing themselves around the process of satisfying customers. First and foremost, he says, they have to be E.T.D.B.W. (*Easy To Do Business With*).

How can dentists be easy to do business with?

Numerous ideas have been discussed: being on time for appointments; available for emergencies; language fluency; a user-friendly

Web site; extended hours to name a few. Here are some additional possibilities:

"I know of practices," says Larry Rosenthal, DDS, New York, NY, "that ask for so much information during the first phone call, they actually drive patients away. Be positive: tell prospective patients how happy you are they called your office."[49]

"I think it's important that you get new patients in the door quickly," says consultant Charles W. Blair, DDS, Charlotte, NC, "not necessarily tomorrow, but within three or four business days. Your broken-appointment rate will be less and it indicates you're committed to the new patient."[50]

Make it easy for patients to ask questions. Many are intimidated, aren't sure how to express their concerns, or are afraid of looking foolish. At the end of an exam, for example, ask patients, "Do you have any other concerns about anything in your mouth?"

Some dentists consider infants and toddlers brought along by parents to be an imposition on their staff and, whenever possible, discourage it. But this makes it difficult for parents who are unable to find (or afford) a baby sitter. Not so at North Gwinnett Dental Care in Sugar Hill, GA, where an onsite childcare area is provided for patients' children at Bridgett Jorgensen, DMD, and Kristin Jorgensen, DDS. "Upon arriving at the practice, they discover a 'dental home' with a warm, inviting living room for the adults and a supervised playroom for children."[51]

Have your staff help patients in any way they can with the determination of their insurance benefits and the filing of the necessary forms. A sign in the staff lounge of one office reads: "Please do not be abusive to patients with insurance problems. They're 75 percent of our practice."

FROM THE SUCCESS FILES

After 40 years of making people stand in line at its parks, Disney woke up and instituted FastPass, which allows visitors to reserve a spot in line and eliminate the wait. An astonishing 95% of its visitors like the change. "We have reinvented how to visit a park," Disney VP Dale Stafford told a reporter. "We have been teaching people how to stand in line since 1955, and now we are telling them they don't have to. Of all the things we can do and the marvels we can create with attractions, this is something that will have profound influence on the entire industry."[52]

REALITY CHECK

"What many companies fail to understand," states an advertorial in *The New York Times*, "is the importance of eliminating complexity and making it easy for the customer to do business with them. It is irrelevant to customers whether they are interacting with a company in person over the phone or on a Web site. They only want to know their needs are being addressed and that the history of the relationship is recognized and understood by the company."[53]

ACTION STEP

Schedule a staff meeting to discuss various ways to make your practice E.T.D.B.W. It will heighten everyone's awareness of this important strategy to differentiate your practice and give it a substantial and sustainable competitive edge.

18 Be consistent

- Does out-of-date equipment imply out-of-date knowledge and skills?
- Does an office that is anything less than meticulously clean cast suspicions on the quality of care?
- Can a receptionist who gives patients a hard time about seeing the doctor in an "emergency" or changing appointments "sour" them against your practice?
- Do aesthetic defects in your and/or your staffs' smiles detract from your credibility?

Perhaps not, but to many people these inconsistencies send negative messages. The reason? People tend to judge the *unknown* by the *known*. As Larry Rosenthal, DDS, New York, NY, has written, "Orange shag carpeting will not sell cosmetic dentistry."[54]

This phenomena emphasizes the need for *consistency* between the image you want your practice to project to others and the image it does project.

If you want to communicate a message of "quality care," then everything in your practice and everything you, your associates and staff members do, must exude *quality*—clearly, compellingly and consistently.

FROM THE SUCCESS FILES

"I learned the hard way," says Robert A. Koetting, OD, FAAO, St. Louis, MO, "that higher rent for the right location is a good investment. When I moved into a high-rise building in an upscale neighborhood, the practice boomed. I realized afterward that I should've done it sooner."[55]

Notes

1. Tenuta CD. What Makes Your Practice Special. *Rehab Economics,* Volume 9, Number 2, 42, March, 2001.
2. Citrin JM, Neff TJ. Doing the Right Things Right. *New York Times,* November 11, 1997, 10.
3. Lavers JR. Market Trends in Dentistry. *Dental Economics,* December 2002, 72-77.
4. Drucker P. *Management Tasks, Responsibilities, Practices.* New York: Harper & Row, 1973.
5. Dickerson WG. Frontdesklessness and the Quality Practice. *Dentistry Today,* March 1993, 85.
6. Dawson PE. Want a Thriving Practice? Concentrate on Clinical Excellence. *Dental Economics,* October 1992, 78-79.
7. Bonner P. Building the Aesthetic Practice. *Dentistry Today,* November 1999, 68-75.
8. Mopper KW. Creative Solutions for Everyday Esthetics. *Dental Practice Report,* June 2000, 46-50.
9. Clinical Research Associates. *CRA Newsletter.* October 2000.
10. Weisman G. Cosmetic Dentistry. *Dental Products Report,* November 2003, 18-26.
11. Garcia A. Just Say Yes to Enhanced Visualization Systems. *Dental Economics.* February 2003, 124-126.
12. Sheets CG, Paquette JM. Enhancing Precision Through Magnification, *Dentistry Today,* January 1998, 44-49.
13. Oral Health in America: A Report of the Surgeon General. *U.S. Department of Health and Human Services,* Executive Summary, 2000.
14. Leonard M. New Techniques for Diagnosis Oral Cancer. *Dental Economics,* June 2000, 126-131.
15. Benjamin SD. Improving Your Bottom Line With Digital Photograph. *Dental Economics,* April 2003, 111-116.
16. Samaras CD. Why Dentists Need Technology. *Contemporary Esthetics and Restorative Practice,* November 2003, 50.
17. Dalin JB. Can You Paradigm? *Dental Economics,* January 2004, 106.
18. Rosenberg S. The Light Fantastic. *Dental Economics,* May 2003, 88-94.
19. Goff S. How Workhorse Systems Are Faring. Dental Products Report, December 2003, 70-76.
20. Antenucci EL. Intraoral Video and Communication Excellence. *The Journal of the New York State Academy of General Dentistry,* March 1995, 8-10.
21. MacFarlane GA. How to Profit from Lasers. *Dental Economics,* March 2003, 76-78.

22. Five Ways to Make Your Web Site a Profitbuilder. *Blair/McGill Advisory,* July 2003, 4.
23. Levato C. Freydberg B. Link Up With Your World. *Dental Practice Report,* Web Guide 2000, 27-30.
24. Farr C. Dentistry Takes the Cybercure: Scheduling, Consultations, Records Move to the Net. *Dentistry Today,* May 2000, 106-112.
25. Hiner S. It's the User Satisfaction, Stupid. *Quirk's Marketing Research Review,* January 2004, 42-44.
26. Osias G. You Have the Cure, So Let Patients Know It. http://www.sightstree.com, accessed April 18, 2001.
27. Make Your Web Site Reach Out to Patients, *Dental Economics,* August 2000, 38, 40, 170.
28 www.dentalpgh.com/lab.htm.
29. Bauer L. The Glorious Benefits of Paperless Dentistry. *Woman Dentist Journal,* March 2004, 32, 34, 67.
30. McDonnell J. The Paperless Office. *Dental Practice Report,* March 2003, 57-58.
31. *Chairside Chatter,* Fall, 2003 Vol. 4.
32. Now's The Time to Invest in Your Practice. *Blair/McGill Advisory,* April 2003, 8.
33. Miles L. *Dynamic Dentistry,* Virginia Beach, VA: Link Publishing, 2003, 33.
34. http://www.atlantacenterforcosmeticdentistry.com/dental/emergency info.jsp
35. *OBG Management,* December 1994
36. www.ianshuman.com.
37. Gailmard N. How Long Do Your Patients Have to Wait? http://www.optometric.com/showtip.asp?tip=96, November 19, 2003.
38. Godin S. *Wisdom, Inc.* New York: HarperBusiness, 1995.
39. Land J. Twenty Rules of the Road. *APMA News,* November 1995, 42, 46.
40. Ousborne AL Jr. Viewpoint. *Dental Economics,* August 2000, 12, 14.
41. Hagerman J. Terrifying, Troublesome or Terrific? *Dentistry Today,* December 2003, 40-43.
42. Armas GC. Surge in Non-English Speaking Households. *San Francisco Chronicle,* October 9 2003, A2.
43. Krauss C. Gay Marriage Plan: Sign of Sweeping Social Change in Canada. *The New York Times,* June 19, 2003.
44. Miller C. Marketing Savvy. *AGD Impact,* April 2004, 17.
45. Scarlett MI. Science News and Resources. *Woman Dentist Journal,* January 2004, 14.
46. Translated Patient Health History Forms. *Dental Editors' Digest,* September 2003.
47. http://www.nsdadentists.com.
48. Mick BA. Your Voices, *Medical Economics,* February 2001, 96.
49. Rosenthal L. A Top 10 List of Mistakes in Practice Management. *Dental Economics,* April 1998.
50. Kehoe B, Blunk D. The New Gold Standard in Patient Service, *Dental Practice & Finance,* January/February 1998, 15-19.
51. Jorgensen B, Jorgensen K, Balancing Act: How to Combine Personal and Professional Living for Pleasure and Profit. *Woman Dentist Journal,* March/April 2003, 46-52.

52. Godin S. If It's Broke, Fix It *Fast Company,* October 2003, 131.
53. Customer Relationships in a Wired World. *The New York Times,* February 14, 2000.
54. Rosenthal L. How to Develop an Esthetic-Centered Practice. *Dental Economics,* January 1997, 26-29.
55. Koetting RA. Unlocking Your Potential. *Optometric Management,* February 2001, 120.

2

Establish an Emotional Connection

What if you could add one element to your strategy for practice growth that would differentiate your practice in a highly meaningful way, make patients more loyal, and ultimately increase your profitability?

And what if it's something so simple, so fundamental, that's it's been there all along, but you and your staff just haven't been able to harness its power?

That element is an *emotional connection* with patients.

Research indicates that strong satisfaction with a product or service, although a prerequisite for loyalty, doesn't guarantee *committed* patients. Something else is required: a bridge between satisfaction and loyalty.

An emotional connection bridges that gap in a way that makes patients feel so valued and cared for, they'll go out of their way to be loyal.

The common thread of the "secrets" in this chapter is that *emotional connection*. Combined with *expertise,* it will differentiate your practice in ways that will be profoundly meaningful and appreciated by your patients.

HARD-LEARNED LESSON

"The emotional realm is where relationships are established and loyalty thrives," say Scott Robinette and Claire Brand in their book, *Emotion Marketing.* "This is where the rest of the marketplace will have a hard time following. This is where the game is won."[1]

19 The relationship-based practice

"The Pankey philosophy is basically centered on a relationship-based approach between the doctor and patient that is fundamental to fee-for-service practices," explains Irwin M. Becker, DDS, Education Chairman of the Pankey Institute. "It is a blend between technical and behavioral excellence. It also has a lot to do with the dentist becoming aware that what he or she is really being compensated for is his/her skill, care and judgment. Thus, this is a movement away from the typical commodity-based approach to dentistry."

"Most dentists start at the Institute," Dr. Becker says, "with the concept that they can provide items that are of use to the patient, such as crowns, bridges, partials and bite splints, and that dentistry is based on an exchange of money for those items. Unlike other areas of the health care field, where managed care has really created more of a pure business climate, our philosophy centers around the belief that the role of the dentist is to contribute skill, care, and judgment that leads to an expert diagnosis rather than simply selling a product. After all, the 'units' of dentistry in which the insurance industry is so interested are really manufactured by the technician in many cases. Our contribution is the brains and experience in design and implementation of an appropriate treatment plan."

"When dentists develop this understanding and relationship with the patient and change the paradigm," Dr. Becker says, "they begin to enjoy the difference this philosophy represents. They are happier and feel better about themselves and their profession. I have seen this happen over and over again in the years I have been involved with the Institute. Using this philosophy, dentists really begin to attract patients who are looking for that exceptional kind of care. It may not be the fastest and cheapest venue, but it is a relationship with their dentist that has depth. It prompts the dentist to allow time to express the compassion and concern that so many patients are looking for today. The result of this style of practice is that as the doctor gets better control of the schedule—not running from patient to patient and room to room—he/she will develop an in-depth relationship with each patient and become more able to achieve optimal care. The optimal care we are talking about leads to much less need for aggressive dental care in future years."[2]

HARD-LEARNED LESSON

In a relationship-based practice, the patient is buying *you*, not "dentistry."

REALITY CHECK

Dearing & Associates conducted a survey of 4957 women who were asked if they would switch physicians if they could not "relate" to their doctor. A total of 89.1 percent (4038) indicated they would find another physician if this situation occurred. Many respondents indicated they had already taken such action.[3]

20 The obvious secret

An *emotional connection* is established when you and your staff demonstrate an interest in a patient as a person and not just as a patient.

FROM THE SUCCESS FILES

"At his office in Bridgeton, NJ, Steve Rasner, DDS, puts a premium on attending skills. He encourages his staff to take notes on patients, memos to themselves about someone's upcoming marriage, say, or vacation to Europe. 'Everyone has to make patients feel valued,' says Dr. Rasner. 'And the way to do that is to know about their lives. So when they sit in the dental chair, you can say 'How did you make out with that surgery last October?' or 'How is your daughter Kelsey doing in her first year of college?' You have to care enough to keep notes. Now that doesn't sound very sophisticated, but it's a reality; it makes people come back to you."[4]

Orthodontist Eric Ploumis, DMD, JD, Larchmont, NY, treats many of the children who attend the nearby French American school and a few years ago, hired a tutor to teach him French. "He did so," reports *The New York Times*, "not to communicate more clearly with his young patients, who are mostly conversant in English. No, Dr. Ploumis also wanted to be able to connect with their mothers."[5]

"My goal," says periodontist Sunie Marchbanks, DDS, Dallas, TX, "is to try to 'wow' every one of my patients—not only by giving them the best patient care, but by giving them emotional care as well."[6]

HARD-LEARNED LESSON

"The level to which you build your practice," says consultant/speaker Paul Homoly, DDS, "is dependent upon your ability to build rapport. To patients, rapport is quality."[7]

REALITY CHECK

In their book *Emotion Marketing,* Scott Robinette and Claire Brand write, "There's an irrefutable business case for showing you care. As it turns out, caring is essential to loyalty."

Hallmark Cards Inc. examined how four variables as defined by its customers—caring, trust, length of patronage, and overall satisfaction—can predict customer loyalty. The Hallmark study found '"caring" to be twice as important to customers as any of the other three variables in predicting loyalty.[8]

21　Empathy is the key

"Empathy," says internationally known clinician Dick Barnes, DDS, "is the key to both understanding and influencing others. Empathy is letting people know you understand what they have said or what they are feeling, or both. If you want to be understood, then you have to understand. You have to have both the right attitude and proper technique to understand the heart and mind of another person."[9]

FROM THE SUCCESS FILES

At the Hunterdon Medical Center in Flemington, NJ, medical residents spend 3 hours learning how it feels to be old. "A makeup artist deepens the lines on their face, adds gray to their hair and powders a pallor onto their skin. They are given yellowed contact lenses with a smearing of Vaseline to blur their vision, they don rubber gloves to dim their sense of touch and they wear wax earplugs to diminish their hearing. Splints are fastened to their joints, making it difficult to move. Raw peas in their shoes simulate corns and calluses."

"With their limitations in place, they are sent to several departments in the hospital. In the X-ray clinic, the residents are sent into small changing rooms and told to undress then redress. At the pharmacy, they are required to fill out Medicaid insurance forms in order to receive a variety of prescriptions. They then return to the program training room where they are assigned a variety of seemingly simple tasks: thread a needle, read the label and open the child-proof caps on the medicine vials, open an orange juice container, unwrap the plastic from a bran muffin."

"In addition to increasing the sensitivity of those who work with the elderly," says Linda F. Bryant, coordinator of the program, "this training has brought visible changes to the hospital. Signs have been made easier to read, registration counters have been lowered to wheelchair height and elevator doors have been altered to allow slower moving patients more time to get on and off."[10]

22 Listen, really listen, to patients

"Your greatest asset to future happiness and success in dentistry," says Irwin M. Becker, DDS, is the time you spend listening to your patients. This pre-clinical and co-discovery examination time is the activity that really differentiates your practice. It is your premier opportunity to personalize your relationship with each patient, forming the basis of a trusting doctor-patient relationship. And it permits you to recognize which patients are ready for complete dentistry and which need to start with Phase 1 care."[11]

Related to spending adequate time with patients and answering questions is the importance of listening to patients in a skillful and understanding way. "It reduces your risk of exposure to malpractice claims," says New York City attorney Andrew Feldman, who often defends healthcare providers in such matters. Among his recommendations:

Pay attention when a patient speaks.

Look like you're paying attention. Looking for example, at a patient's chart or worse, your watch, implies less-than-total interest on your part. Someone worth listening *to* is worth looking *at*.

Get involved while listening. Don't be a deadpan. Lean forward. Nod your head as the patient speaks. Respond to the patient's cues and facial expressions. Periodically say "uh-huh," "that's interesting," or other words to show you're listening.

Paraphrase or summarize what you've understood the patient to have said. It lets patients know you've correctly heard the message. And if you haven't, it will enable you and the patient to achieve clarity. Such responses are time-consuming but help ensure that two-way communication takes place.

And finally, before concluding the patient's visit, always ask: "Is there anything else you would like to ask me?"

"This dialoging back and forth," Mr. Feldman says, "is important, not only for its clinical significance, but also as a secondary benefit, a means to minimize your exposure to malpractice claims."

FROM THE SUCCESS FILES

"Effective listening is the single most important element in a successful consultation," says Jeffrey Golub-Evans, DDS, FAACD, New York, NY. "If you're not listening, you may be discussing the wrong service entirely. If you're not listening, you may be contributing to a patient's sense that you are not interested, not concerned, not compassionate, and maybe not even competent. Get it? Shut up and listen."[12]

---

23 Follow-up phone calls

Follow-up phone calls to patients following an emergency or surgery produce a powerful emotional connection. They may also have clinical significance.

ACTION STEP

Such calls can be made from the office (between patients), from a car phone, or from your home. They need not be time-consuming.

Explain the purpose of the call by saying at the start, "I'm just between appointments (or "on my way home" or "about to sit down to dinner"), and I was thinking of you. How are you feeling?"

Occasionally, patients have discomfort that they had not expected or, perhaps, more discomfort than they expected, along with varying degrees of concern about what this discomfort means.

The situation may just call for reassurance, a reminder of previously given home-care instructions, an adjustment in medication, or other special instructions depending on the symptoms.

In such cases, there's an opportunity to turn even this highly positive emotional connection into a *truly memorable* one, by telephoning an anxious patient a *second time* later the same day or evening to see whether the home-care instructions, medication, or just the passage of time has improved the situation.

Follow-up phone calls occasionally uncover situations that require further attention. More frequently, they give patients "peace of mind" about what they're experiencing and evidence your genuine interest in them.

FROM THE SUCCESS FILES

"Calling patients the night of their surgery," says periodontist Douglas M. Neuman, DMD, Lexington, KY, "is still the single, most talked about thing we do."

24 Be "likable"

Another common trait among high-performance dentists is that they tend to be *likable*. What a difference it makes in the rhythm of the office, the image of the practice, patient satisfaction, and everyone's "mood" at the end of the day.

A likable personality is a priceless asset (some say "necessity") in any service occupation, dentistry included. But it's frequently underestimated by dentists convinced that knowledge and skills are all that matter.

What is a "likable personality?" Bobbie Gee, former image and appearance coordinator for Disneyland, says likable people:

- Smile easily
- Have a good sense of humor
- Are great listeners
- Know common sense etiquette and use it
- Compliment easily and often
- Are self-confident
- Engage you in conversation about yourself
- Can laugh at themselves
- Are approachable[13]

25 Have fun

"The last thing people expect in a dental office," says Paul Homoly, DDS, "is a pleasant experience. Having fun means surrounding yourself with energetic, humorous people. If you're not having fun, I guarantee your patients aren't. Lighten up—dentistry is not life or death. Patients will love you and your staff when they sense you love what you do and are fun to be with."[14]

At the Long Beach, NY, office of South Nassau Dermatology, a sign at the receptionist's desk had everyone chuckling:

> If You Are Grouchy, Irritable,
> Or Just Plain Mean, There
> Will Be A $10 Charge For
> Putting Up With You

HARD-LEARNED LESSON

"Try to make working at Ogilvy & Mather fun," said famed advertising man David Ogilvy, founder of the world-renowned agency that bears his name. "When people aren't having any fun, they seldom produce good advertising. Kill grimness with laughter. Encourage exuberance. Get rid of sad dogs who spread gloom."[15]

26 The little things that cost the least, which count the most

Most dentists agree that *loyal patients* deserve preferential treatment. What many dentists and particularly their staffs may not realize is that people who are loyal to a service provider *fully expect* preferential treatment, whether it's dentist or a bank.

Here's some market research to prove the point.

People feel strongly about being treated as a preferred customer when visiting a branch of a financial institution, according to a research study by Atlanta-based Synergistics Research Corporation. Consumers were asked to rate their level of agreement with the statement, *"When I do a lot of business with a particular bank, it is important to me to be treated like a preferred customer."*

Nearly eight in ten "strongly" agreed with this statement. Another one in six "somewhat" agreed, making overall agreement with this statement almost unanimous.

These findings were based on a telephone survey of 1041 consumers age 18 or older with household incomes of more than $25,000. The sample also included 201 individuals with household incomes of more than $100,000.

"These findings," says Genie M. Driskill, COO of Synergistics, "indicate it may be the little things that cost the least, which count the most."[16]

What is "preferential treatment?" Whether it's a bank or a dentist's office, it's an environment that makes people feel special. It's remembering patients' names and pronouncing them correctly. It's maintaining eye contact when talking with them. It's coming in early or staying late as a special accommodation for a loyal patient for whom an appointment time is not available. It's returning their phone calls as quickly as possible. It's knowing patients' likes and dislikes and catering to them.

Above all, it takes *teamwork* on everyone's part to make an emotional connection happen, and that connection will result in high patient retention.

ACTION STEP
Schedule a staff meeting to discuss the kinds of preferential treatment that would be most meaningful to your loyal patients. This discussion alone will get everyone rowing in the same direction.

27 Address patients' special needs

While conducting an in-service program for Rehabilitation Associates, Inc., in Mequon, WI, I was shown a self-assessment form given to patients on the day of their visits for occupational therapy. Patients were asked to place an "X' next to the words that best describe their feelings on that day. The heading was "Today I Feel," and among the words on the list of 35 were happy, apprehensive, frustrated, quiet, hostile, nervous, impatient, disinterested, friendly, and worthless.

REALITY CHECK
Imagine how much easier it is to relate to a patient and establish an emotional connection when you know his or her state of mind at the time.

FROM THE SUCCESS FILES
On the home page of the Web site of Thomas K. Hedge, DDS, West Chester, OH, is the following message: "Do You Have Special Needs or Concerns? Let Us Know By Clicking Here." The link then takes the patient to the following page[17]:

The Dental Health Center
Thomas K. Hedge, DDS

Handle Me With Care

First Name	M.I.	Last Name

☐ I gag easily.

☐ I feel out of control when I'm lying down in the dental chair.

☐ I have not been to the dentist for a long time, and I feel uncomfortable about what you will say about my teeth and dental hygiene.

☐ Pain relief is a top priority for me.

☐ I don't like shots (or I've had a bad reaction to shots).

☐ Please tell me what I need to know about my mouth in order to make an informed decision.

☐ My teeth are very sensitive.

☐ I don't like the sound of the tool that makes picking and scraping noise.

☐ I don't like cotton in my mouth.

☐ I hate the noise of the drill.

☐ Please respect my time. I don't want to be left sitting.

☐ I want to know the cost up front. No money surprises please.

☐ I have difficulty listening and remembering what I hear when sitting in a dental chair.

☐ I have health problems and questions that we need to discuss.

Submit

Patients whose needs and preferences have been overlooked by previous dentists greatly appreciate the thoughtfulness expressed by this questionnaire.

28 Create a calming environment

Anxious patients tend to be more fidgety, complaining, and difficult to treat, and their behavior tends to increase the level of stress for everyone in the office.

FROM THE SUCCESS FILES

"To help ease patient anxieties," says Debra Gray King, DDS, FAACD, president of the Atlanta Center for Cosmetic Dentistry, "we have taken a whole-office approach to creating a soothing, peaceful atmosphere. Unlike the typical sterile feel and smell of most dental offices, we have tried to create an ambiance reminiscent of a fine, upscale resort. The reception area is accented with comfortable furnishings, flowers, oil paintings, and a refreshment center with coffee, tea, bottled water, juice and cookies fresh-baked on-site. This immediately tends to relax patients anticipating a dental visit. Instead of assistants in scrubs, cheerful dental concierges dressed in designer outfits greet patients by name. The gentler, softer tone and surroundings go a long way to calm patients' fears."[18]

29 Be child-friendly

The following form, given to me by Steve Randell, DDS, MS, is used by the Department of Dentistry at the Illinois Masonic Medical Center in Chicago. It is sent to parents in advance of a child's first visit. The brief introduction explains its one and only purpose.

Pre-Need Questionnaire For Children

The purpose of this questionnaire is to learn more about your child before beginning his/her

dental care. Your answers will help to make your child's visits to the dentist more predictable and

productive.

1) Is this your child's first visit to a dental office? Yes___   No ___

2) If not, how would you describe your child's previous visits _____

_____

3) How long is your child's attention span at home (other than TV watching?) _____

_____

4) Does your child have any pets, hobbies, special interests or recent accomplishments? If yes,

please list _____

_____

5) Is there any additional information that might help us in treating your child? _____

_____

QUESTIONS TO CONSIDER

- Would the information from such a questionnaire help (as the form says) to make a child's first visit "more predictable and productive?"
- What impression do you think this pre-need questionnaire would make on the parent(s) receiving it prior to the child's first visit?
- Does it convey a "child-friendly" image?
- Would the information obtained by the questionnaire enable you and your staff to establish an emotional connection with the child?

FROM THE SUCCESS FILES

Separate waiting areas for adults and children in the award-winning Really Smile Dental office of Rod Strickland, DDS, and Dave Smith, DDS, in Fishers, IN, "cater to their unique sensibilities," writes Barbara Baccei. "The children's area features a captivating 1000-gallon salt water aquarium, toy furniture, colorful books, and a 43 inch DVD television with shows for kids. In the adult area, patients lounge on soft leather sofas and chairs, have their own 43 inch television tuned for patient education, and a workstation with a computer and telephone."[19]

30 Provide your patients a service you hope they never have to use

One of the greatest fears of parents today is that their child will get lost, or worse, be abducted. A couple of dollars and a few minutes of chair time is a small investment to make for a huge return of being able to assist authorities in tracking a missing child or making a positive identification. Few children have fingerprints taken and the successful fight against tooth decay has left many children with no cavities and few dental records.

Toothprints® bite impressions, developed by pedodontist David A. Tesini, DMD, MS, Natick, MA, are a simple, cost-effective way of documenting a child's unique dental characteristics showing the size and shape of the teeth, position of the teeth within the dental arch, and the relationship of the maxillary and mandibular arches to each other.

The arch-shaped thermoplastic wafer also captures saliva, a powerful source of human scent, and a DNA sample. The completed tooth print is then sealed in a zipper type bag and given to the parent to take home for safekeeping.

Many dentists have begun tooth printing in their offices," writes Joseph Blaes, DDS, editor of *Dental Economics*. "They take the prints at ages 3, 7 and 13. It is an easy technique and can be done by any member of the dental team. Parents love the program and praise it highly."[20]

Most dentists who offer this service do so at no charge to their patients as a community service. Some offer on their Web sites to provide this service to any resident of their community. Others do so at local health fairs. Many, like Jack Von Bulow, DDS, Temple City, CA, have joined other dentists to provide Toothprints to fourth graders in local school districts.

Howard Glaser, DDS, FAGD, FAAFS, a forensic dentist in Fort Lee, NJ, says "Toothprints are a valuable adjunctive aid in helping to formulate the identification of an individual of any age."[21]

Toothprint kits with 25 or 100 wafers in both child and adult sizes along with storage bags can be ordered from SDS Kerr authorized dealers. For more information, visit www.kerrdental.com.

"This is a wonderful program for your office," says Dr. Blaes, "and your staff will be proud to participate."

31 Be senior-friendly

"America is going gray," say authors Elizabeth Vierck and Kris Vierck. "Today 1 in 8 Americans are 65 or older, and by 2020 it is expected that 1 in 6 will be in that age group. From 2010 to 2050, the senior population is expected to more than double from 40 million to 82 million."[22]

REALITY CHECK

"If your practice targets an older demographic group, don't discount the Web," says John McDonnell, special reports Web editor for *Dental Practice Report*. "The UCLA Internet Report, 'Surveying the Digital Future,' shows that Internet users span every age group, with 64 percent of 56-60 year-olds reporting access to the Internet and 72 percent of 46-55 year-olds now using the Internet."[23]

FROM THE SUCCESS FILES

On the office Web site of Lynn Carlisle, DDS, Fort Collins, CO, is the following announcement that certainly makes an emotional connection:

Dentistry for Seniors
"We are seniors who enjoy working with seniors. We have a special niche in our practice for seniors. This niche is because of the length of time we have been practicing and our interest in working with people who have passed midlife."

"We enjoy talking about grandkids—our team has three—and the stories about this time of life. We also have extensive experience in solving the dental problems of this stage of life. We have a web page for seniors. Click on the patient education button to the left—then click on seniors."[24]

32 Address the needs of deaf/hard-of-hearing patients

There are between 22 and 24 million Americans who are deaf/hard-of-hearing. Some have relatively minor difficulty in hearing. Others are profoundly deaf and communicate with sign language, lip reading, written messages, or a combination of these methods.

Recognizing this need, Christopher D. Sullivan, III, manager of special needs financial services at Merrill Lynch, established the first Deaf/Hard of Hearing Investor Service on Wall Street to provide telecommunication access for the deaf, sign language interpreters, closed caption videotapes, and hiring of deaf financial advisors.[25]

FROM THE SUCCESS FILES

Beverly B. Miller, OD, has built a specialty practice in the Washington, D.C. area by addressing the needs of deaf and hard-of-hearing patients.

This area has a greater density of such patients than do many other parts of the country, in part because of nearby Gallaudet University for the deaf and hard-of-hearing and partly because of the great number of federal government employees who are deaf or hard-of-hearing.

The first step, says Dr. Miller, is to become fluent in sign language. "Luckily," she adds, "I was motivated because I have some deaf acquaintances."

Step two is to make your practice accessible to deaf and hard-of-hearing patients. They have to be able to call in and make their own appointments and your staff has to be comfortable with this. Filling this need requires installation of a Telecommunications Device for the Deaf (TDD) in your office so patients can call and then type in their messages. In addition, Dr. Miller has offered courses in signing to her staff.

Step three is to get the word out. In the beginning, Dr. Miller spent most of her evenings for about a year giving lectures on general vision care to student groups at nearby Gallaudet University as well as groups at Gallaudet's high school and elementary program. She also alerted local school nurses to the special services she could provide deaf and hard-of-hearing patients.

33 A friendly staff

One of the first things patients notice about a practice is the *ambiance*.

An upbeat, friendly staff is a huge plus for a practice, especially in today's impersonal, "sign in, sit down, shut up" healthcare environment. And it's never an accident.

Friendliness is usually easy to spot. One of the signs is the number of times a job candidate *smiles* during the interview.

"Nordstrom, the retailer based in Seattle, is famous for its friendly employees, but no special program made them that way. 'When companies ask us if we'd like to come out and talk about our program, we just don't have a lot to say,' a spokeswoman, Brooke White said. 'There's no great science to this. Mostly, we just think we're making good hiring decisions.'"[26]

34 The secret of the Philadelphia hoagie

Reminiscing about his early life in Philadelphia, Joel Novack, DPM (now practicing in Cleveland, OH) recalled the sensational hoagies (hero) sandwiches made by a local chain of delicatessens. On one occasion, he asked the proprietor what made their hoagies so much better than those made by other delis.

"Is it the crusty bread?" Dr. Novack asked.

"No," the proprietor replied.

"Is it the special meats and cheeses?"

Again, the answer was "no."

"How about the olive oil? The condiments?"

"No," the proprietor said, "It's *everything*."

"That simple lesson," Dr. Novack says, "made a lasting impression. And years later, I realized the same principle applies to practice. It's no one thing that leads to success. It's *everything*—starting from the moment the patient first calls the office. It's how they're spoken to by staff members and doctors, how their concerns are addressed, or how their insurance coverage is handled. It's whether patients see signs of competence and caring during their office visit or an assembly-line attitude. It's whether they see a neat, spotlessly clean, well-equipped office or something less."

True differentiation in an endeavor seldom results from doing just one thing that much better than anyone else. *It comes from doing 100 things just one percent better.*

REALITY CHECK

"I often advise businesspeople (and businesses)" says author and business visionary Tom Peters, "to describe how they are special in 25 words or less—what makes them stand out from the 'me too' herd. If they can't do that, they ought to pack it up."[27]

Notes

1. Robinette S, Brand C, Lenz V. *Emotion Marketing*. New York: McGraw-Hill, 2001.
2. Bonner P. The Pankey Institute Enters the New Millennium. *Dentistry Today,* January 2000, 40-45, 64, used with permission of Irwin M. Becker, DDS.
3. Dearing RH, Gordon HA, Sohner DM et al. *Marketing Women's Health Care.* New York: Aspen Publishers Inc., 1987.
4. McCann D. Satisfaction Not Guaranteed. *Dental Practice Report,* July/August 2001, 31-34.
5. Mohn T. All Aboard the Foreign Language Express. *The New York Times,* October 11, 2000.
6. Marchbanks S. A Twist on Pain Reduction. *Woman Dentist Journal,* April 2004, 8, 10-11.
7. Homoly P. The Day of Awakening, *Dental Economics,* January 1998.
8. Robinette S. Brand C, Lenz V. *Emotion Marketing.* New York: McGraw-Hill, 2001.
9. Barnes D. Why Using Empathy Can Lead to Greater Case Acceptance. *Dental Products Report,* October 1998, 134-129.
10. Murray K. Make Nice and Make It Snappy: Companies Try Courtesy Training. *The New York Times,* April 2, 1995.
11. Becker IM. Building a Five-Star Practice. *California Dental Association Journal,* April 1995.
12. Golub-Evans J. The Comfort Zone: Looking & Listening for Better Patient Care and Communication. *Dental Products Report,* October 1997, 34-38.
13. Gee B. *Creating a Million Dollar Image for Your Business; Smart Strategies for Building an Image That Works.* Berkeley, CA: Pagemill Press, 1966.
14. Homoly P. The Dentist's Dozen: Great Ways to Build Value Before You Recommend Care. www.paulhomoly.com.
15. Ogilvy D. Blood, Brains & Beer. New York: Atheneum, 1978.
16. The Customer is King—or, at Least Wants to Be Treated Royally at the Ranch. http://www.synergisticsresearch.com.
17. http://www.dentalhealthcenter.com.

18. King DG. Is Spa Dentistry Going Mainstream? *Woman Dentist Journal,* January 2004, 8-12.
19. Baccei B. How a Building Can 'Really Smile.' *Dental Economics,* April 2000, 64-74.
20. Blaes J. Impressive! *Dental Economics,* February 2003, 162, 174.
21. Personal communication.
22. Vierck E, Hodges K. *Aging: Demographics, Health, and Heallth Services.* Westport, CT: Greenwood Press, 2003.
23. McDonnell J. New UCLA Survey Reveals Benefit of the Web. *Dental Practice Report,* March 2003, 62.
24. http://www.carlisledds.com.
25. Ellin A. Helping Deaf Investors, *The New York Times,* December 7, 2003, BU 11.
26. Murray K. Make Nice and Make It Snappy: Companies Try Courtesy Training, *The New York Times,* April 2, 1995, Section 3.
27. Peters T. *The Pursuit of Wow!* New York: Vintage Books, 1994.

3

Take Your Practice to the Next Level: Make It a "Brand"

"Today's consumers are increasingly brand-centric," reports the trade magazine *Hotels,* "and marketers know creating a strong brand identity is a great way to differentiate their product and build customer loyalty."[1]

35 Brand your practice

Your brand represents the feelings that you and your practice evoke in the minds of patients, colleagues, physicians, and other potential referral sources. It's who they think you are. It's what you stand for: the expertise, quality of care, service, integrity, and professionalism that others associate with you. It's also the type of mental awareness that predisposes patients to choose your practice over others.

If you are fortunate enough to have what's called "*top-of-mind*" status, it will be your practice patients first think of when they need a dentist (or orthodontist, periodontist, or other specialist).

People buy branded consumer products from computers to cars, expecting a level of quality, service, reliability, and satisfaction. If those expectations are met, people buy again. That's "brand loyalty." If the brand doesn't live up to expectations, buyers simply go elsewhere.

44

A practice brand works the same way. Every minute of every day, it broadcasts information about *who* you are, *what* you and your staff do, and *how* you do it. If your brand is sending out the right messages about what people can expect when they're in your office, they will travel farther, wait longer, pay more, make more referrals, *and* remain more loyal.

"Your brand," says consultant Andrea T. Eliscu, RN, "is your personality. It can be a name, design or symbol which enhances the value of your practice beyond its functional purpose—something that distinguishes it from others. A strong brand makes a promise. A strong brand is trustworthy and possesses great value. It has meaning, prestige, and presence, and it helps confirm what is expected."[2]

Over time, the added value that accrues from branding is referred to as *brand equity.* It includes such benefits to your practice as consumer awareness, perceived quality, and patient loyalty.

ACTION STEP

"Start by identifying the qualities or characteristics that make you distinctive from your colleagues," says author/speaker Tom Peters (who is himself a brand name as an authority on the new economy). "What have you done lately, this week, to make yourself stand out? What would your colleagues or your patients say is your greatest and clearest strength? Your most noteworthy personal trait?"

"Ask yourself: What do I do that I am most proud of? What have I accomplished that I can unabashedly brag about? If you're going to be a brand," says Peters, "you've got to become relentlessly focused on what you do that adds value, that you're proud of, and most important, that you can shamelessly take credit for."[3]

---

36 Determine the core values of your practice

The next step in developing a brand for your practice is to determine the core values of your practice. Core values are the building blocks of a personal brand and represent what's truly important in your practice: the guiding principles for you and your staff, and the qualities that give it a distinctive character and differentiate it from other practices.

REALITY CHECK

At your next staff meeting, ask each person to write his or her answer to the question: *What's important here?* If it's the first time the subject has been discussed, be prepared for a wide range of answers. Discuss them all and reach a consensus. It could be the most important staff meeting you've ever held.

"Visionary companies tend to have only a few core values, usually between three and six," say consultants James C. Collins and Jerry I. Porras, authors of *Built to Last: Successful Habits of Visionary Companies.* "And indeed, we should expect this, for only a few values can be truly *core*—values so fundamental and deeply held that they will change or be compromised seldom, if ever."

For example, the core values at McDonald's are summarized in the four letters originally conceived by founder Ray Kroc and his earliest franchisers: QSCV (quality, service, cleanliness, and value). These are the guiding principles for all of McDonald's corporate strategies and organizational practices.

"How can we be sure," ask Collins and Porras, "that the core ideologies of highly visionary organizations represent more than just a bunch of nice-sounding platitudes—words with no bite, words meant merely to pacify, manipulate or mislead? We have two answers. First, social psychology research strongly indicates that when people publicly espouse a particular point of view, they become much more likely to behave consistent with that point of view even if they did not previously hold that point of view. Second and more important, the visionary organizations don't merely declare an ideology; they take steps to make the ideology pervasive throughout the organization."[4]

"Passion is a pretty foolproof test of whether a value is a core value," says Mike Moser, who has won over 300 national and international marketing awards. "It will help you include your heart in the decision-making process instead of just your head. Passion is what creates an emotional connection that transcends ads, public relations, brochures, or any other crafted messages that a company puts out."[5]

37 Choose your brand identity

"To help choose your brand identity," says consultant David Schwab, PhD, "do a group exercise with your dental team. Write down as many positive adjectives to describe the practice as your team can think of in a 10 minute brainstorming session. Then go through the list and rate each one on a scale of 1 to 10. Keep the highest-scoring adjectives and discard the rest. Then, continue to rank and prioritize until you have three to five adjectives that you want to use to describe and define the practice. Once this is done, you will have a brand identity, and the staff will have the words they need to communicate your brand to patients and potential patients."[6]

The narrowing of your core values to just a few words works extremely well. The fewer values you and your staff concentrate on, the more focused your practice and the easier the decisions for everyone involved with your brand.

FROM THE SUCCESS FILES

"One's staff and associates should believe in delivering the finest quality dentistry with the best service available," says Larry Rosenthal, DDS, New York, NY, founder and head of the New York Group for Aesthetic and Restorative Dentistry. "Our philosophy is 'Five Star service. Five Star product.'"[7]

"I urge you to examine your practice and determine if it functions in a manner consistent with your most deeply held beliefs and values," says John A. Wilde, DDS, Keokuk, IA. "If it does, you're experiencing a lot of joy. If it doesn't, everyone involved feels the stress that occurs when behaviors aren't consistent with values."[8]

"The staff also has to buy into and own the practice philosophy," says Ronald Jackson, DDS, Middleburg, VA. "The reason there has to be consistent communication of the philosophy, with no contradictions sensed by patients, is that patients today are simply too sharp. If they sense that any staff member doesn't wholeheartedly believe in the dentistry provided in the office, they won't have procedures done."[9]

REALITY CHECK

If excellence, for example, is a core value, then it has to permeate the whole culture of your practice. Core values should live in the world of black and white, not shades of gray. When your core values are black and white, then everyone in your practice understands what's expected of them and you're much closer to doing what you say you're going to do 100% of the time.

38 Brand personality

Every dental practice has a personality. It's impossible for a practice not to have a personality, just as it's impossible for a person not to have a personality. Even "zero" personality is a personality.

Many dental practices, however, fall into that "zero' personality trap. The reason? There is no thought of what the brand personality of the practice should be, so everyone just does his or her own thing. As a result, every interaction with patients takes on the personality of the dentist or team member involved. The brand personality of the practice thus becomes a hodgepodge of various traits that sends mixed messages to patients.

In *Building Strong Brands*, David A. Aaker, Professor of Marketing Strategy at the University of California at Berkeley, talks about a brand personality containing such characteristics as gender (Virginia Slims, female; Marlboro, male), age (Apple, young IBM, older), socioeconomic class (After Eight mints, upscale; Butterfinger, blue-collar), and other classic traits such as warmth, concern, and sentimentality.[10]

ACTION STEP

Schedule a staff meeting to discuss what personality is most appropriate for your practice and the patients you serve. What message are you trying to send? The following questions may help get you started.

Is your practice brand male, female, or neither?
Is your practice brand young, middle-aged, old, or for all ages?
Is your practice brand upscale or blue-collar?
Is your practice brand sophisticated? Mainstream? Down-Home?
Is your practice brand no-nonsense or relaxed and easy-going?

WHY IT MATTERS

Your practice's brand personality, if it is to be consistent, will influence everything about your practice: its location; the colors and decor of your office; the ambiance; artwork; the in-office music system; magazines; stationary and business cards; the practice Web site; the practice brochure; attire of everyone in the office; the personality of the people you hire; and, perhaps most important, the day-to-day interactions that you and your staff have with patients.

39 Brand relevance

The most effective way to go about building a strong personal brand is to make sure your brand resonates and is relevant in the most distinctive way possible for those patients with whom you want to build strong relationships on a long-term basis.

"Building relevance involves a skill that requires reverse thinking," say David McNally and Karl D. Speak, authors of *Be Your Own Brand.* "To be relevant to others, you must move out of your world into theirs. In other words, you first have to determine your patients' needs and interests. Then connect those needs and interests to your own personal strengths and abilities."

"That means relevance is a process," say McNally and Speak. "It starts with questions: What do *they* want? What do *they* need? What do *they* value? What do *they* expect?"

When you have a sense of your patients' needs and their frame of reference, that information can guide your actions in ways that will make your practice relevant.

ACTION STEP

Determine your target population.

"Our commitment to pleasing our guests," states the Target Corporation Annual Report, "is inherent in our strategy: it drives our merchandising as well as many of our investment and operating decisions. As a result, we strongly believe that we need to know our guest and understand her preferences. Though we recognize and respect the individuality of each guest, our research suggests that more than 90 percent of our guests are female with a median age of 45 years. Approximately one-half have earned a college degree and about 40 percent have school-age children at home. By continuing to supplement this guest profile, we are better able to satisfy each guest's wants and needs."[12]

DENTAL DEMOGRAPHICS

"Women account for 86 percent of dental appointments made and are the healthcare decision-makers in the typical household," says Jeffrey B. Dalin, DDS, FACD, FAGD, St. Louis, MO.[13]

"87 percent of all cosmetic procedures," says William Dorfman, DDS, Los Angeles, CA, "are performed on female patients. Women in their 40s to early 70s make the best candidates."[14]

40 Communicate with color

"Colors instantly communicate certain messages about your brand," says Mike Moser, author of *United We Brand*. Because of this instinctive response, it's important to determine whether your office colors are helping or hurting the effectiveness of the messages you want to communicate about your practice.

"Some of the questions you'll want to address," Moser says, "involve the level of sophistication of the colors, and whether the colors elicit the right emotional response. For example, simple colors are the primary and secondary colors on the color wheel (red, yellow, blue, orange, green, and purple). Sophisticated colors are all the other colors (taupe, mauve, sea green, slate blue, maroon, pumpkin, sage, etc)."

"Simple colors tend to be more vibrant and shout louder than sophisticated colors. Toys 'R' Us uses simple colors. Traffic signs around the world use simple colors to stand out along the highway."

"Brands like Armani, Tiffany, and Jaguar on the other hand, use sophisticated colors. The colors communicate a certain understated elegance and, in many ways, set up the expectations of a quieter, more intimate conversation. The rich colors of Starbucks shops create a much different coffee experience from that represented by the simple colors of McDonald's."[15]

REALITY CHECK

Pat Brillo, a consultant for Color Services & Associates in Huntley, IL, stresses that "Selecting the right color is about audience. Who's your audience? What's the message? Just picking a trendy color is not the answer. Different consumers are affected different ways by that color, and trends are constantly changing."[16]

41 The Mayo Clinic

One of the best-known, most highly regarded brand names in healthcare is that of the Mayo Clinic.

"The Mayo name is so famous that it's recognized by 85 percent of Americans," writes Paul Roberts in *Fast Company*. "Patients who walk into the Mayo Clinic in Rochester, MN, enter an environment of comfort and tradition that is worlds apart from the institutional atmosphere of many hospitals. Fine art hangs on walls throughout the clinic. In the waiting areas of each medical department, professional greeters ease new patients through the admission process, reassuring them in homey, upper-midwestern accents. They greet returning patients by name. Doctors see patients in private offices, cozy spaces decorated with personal items, rather than in sterile white-and-chrome exam rooms. The overall effect is one of orderliness, function and above all, vigor."[17]

42 Achieve visibility + credibility

The next step in building your brand is to achieve both visibility and credibility.

Visibility refers to how *well-known* you are in your community. Credibility refers to how *well-regarded and respected* you are. There are four basic permutations.

- **High visibility/high credibility:** This translates into being both well-known and well-regarded. It's obviously the most desirable brand image—the one with the highest potential for attracting new patients. If you've got this image, keep on doing what you have been doing.
- **Low visibility/high credibility:** You're well-regarded and respected but not well-known. The challenge? Increase your visibility in the community so more people become aware of your practice.
- There are countless ways to enhance your visibility. Teach a class at a community college or adult education program. Contribute a column or an opinion piece to your local newspaper. Get involved as a sponsor, organizer, or even founder of charity or civic events such as community theater or Little League.

ACTION STEP

"February is the month for children's dental health," says Lori Trost, DMD, editor of *Woman Dentist Journal*. "What a great opportunity to visit preschools, day-care centers, and elementary schools. Set the stage with videos, handouts, coloring pages, and office tours. Further share your message with stickers, timers, floss, and toothbrushes. This is a wonderful chance to promote your practice and gently impact a new generation of patients."[18]

FROM THE SUCCESS FILES

Scott Coleman, DDS, FAGD, is the "official dentist" to three of the leading theater companies in Houston, TX. Over the years he has created special dental effects for numerous plays from Shakespeare to Dracula.

As a result of his involvement with these theaters, which Dr. Coleman has always enjoyed, he receives prominent mention in the printed program, opening night tickets for himself and his staff, and important name recognition among the actors, production people, and season ticket holders, many of whom have become his patients.

HARD-LEARNED LESSON

Visibility has a funny way of multiplying. The hardest part is getting started.

- **Low visibility/low credibility:** If you're new in practice or have recently moved to a new community, you're most likely unknown.

Resist the temptation to jumpstart your practice with 'tack
tising or aggressive self-promotion that may get you knov
the process *undermine* your credibility and turn off potentia. patients
as well as colleagues, physicians, and other referral sources.

There's a thin line between getting yourself known and promoting
yourself to the point of overkill. But the line is hard to define, because
the level of acceptance is in the mind of the person you're trying to
reach.

"Tacky" works fine for some people. They may even be attracted
to your panache. But in general, our market research shows that for
today's more discerning, Internet-savvy consumers, promotional give-
aways, direct mail, and advertising are far less effective than seeing a
dentist in print as an author or quoted source, attending a talk given
by a dentist, or seeing him or her interviewed on TV.

But even these very effective opportunities to "showcase" your
expertise and professional demeanor can erode credibility if the focus
is on "me, me, me," rather than giving the audience solid, useful
information.

REALITY CHECK

"A key finding of our studies is that advertising is not nearly as
powerful a tool for creating visibility as it once was," says Charles J.
Fombrun, Professor Emeritus of Management at the Stern School of
Business, New York University and Executive Director of the Reputation Institute, a private research group. "A company's name recognition is more credibly and cheaply built through earned media coverage
than through paid promotion."[19]

- **High visibility/low credibility.** This is the worst of the four possibilities. You're well-known but not well-regarded. It's been called
  the "Amtrak Syndrome." The good news: Recovery is possible.
  You need however, to tread carefully and not expect overnight
  results.

HARD-LEARNED LESSON

Never confuse name recognition with brand strength.

ACTION STEP

Take an objective look at what you're doing to "promote" your practice. How well do these efforts meet the visibility/credibility test?

It's an analysis that will help you make the right decision for your practice.

REALITY CHECK

Everything about your practice, and everything you and your staff do and say, communicates credibility (or the lack of it). The way your staff handles phone conversations, the appearance of your office and Web site, and the way you interact with patients are part of the larger message you're sending about your practice.

43 Public speaking

Public speaking, whether you are speaking to study clubs, professional associations, or community groups, is one of the most effective ways of achieving both visibility and credibility. Dentists who do it tend to have *better* practices than those who don't. They're better known. more highly regarded, and they get more new patients.

How does one get started? The average dentist has all the qualifications and ability he or she needs to become an effective public speaker. It's really just an extension of in office patient education.

FROM THE SUCCESS FILES

"One of the things I did to help give exposure to the field of aesthetic and cosmetic dentistry in my community," says author/speaker Ross W. Nash, DDS, Charlotte, NC, "was to begin giving community talks. I went to the public library, found a list of civic organizations and wrote letters to the program chairpersons. I informed them that I would give a presentation about aesthetics in dentistry for a lunch or dinner meeting."

"I began to get numerous invitations and gave several dozen talks in the first few years. The presentations were simply before-and-after slides to illustrate possibilities and a discussion about material and treatment expectations."

"I was always careful," says Dr. Nash, "to talk about what dentistry can offer rather than what 'Ross Nash' can offer. I believe a professional approach rather than a sales approach attracts patients of the highest caliber and speaks well of our profession."[20]

HARD-LEARNED LESSON

The dentist whose only motive for public speaking is to *obtain new patients* will come across as self-serving and leave a negative impression. To avoid any misinterpretation of your motives, make little or no reference to your practice as such, your years of experience, expertise, or patients. Keep it informative and *low-key*. The idea is to establish yourself as an "authority," not as someone who is "looking for business."

ACTION STEP

"Establish yourself as an authority on infant dental care by addressing parents attending prenatal classes at your local hospital," suggests author/coach Steven Schwartz, DDS. "Arrange for presentations for parent support groups at nursery schools and day care centers especially if a pediatric dentist is not providing such a service."[21]

FROM THE SUCCESS FILES

Once a year, Andrew Doerfler, DDS, Spring, TX, gives talks to school children (K-5) using magic to hold the children's attention and help explain the three reasons they should brush and floss their teeth (avoid cavities, bad breath, and gum disease). The children enjoy and learn from his presentations. The teachers and parents are highly pleased with the message, and Dr. Doerfler benefits in more ways than one.

44 Community involvement

"Interestingly, many consumers today are not only looking to invest personal energy in their communities," reports the Yankelovich Monitor®, "but they are also looking to do business with companies that share their dedication to their local area.

"The bottom line: Getting involved at a local level and showing you share an appreciation of community can not only forge a bond with consumers but can also get them talking about your brand."[22]

"Your involvement as a member of the community," says author/ coach Steven Schwartz, DDS, "is always appreciated. Types of activities for which you can volunteer include:

"Sponsor scholarship programs to students interested in entering the dental profession."

"Volunteer your resources to shelters, food banks, hospitals, rescue squads, senior citizens, and child care centers. You don't have to limit your volunteerism to your dental skills. Many of these organizations need individuals to run their daily activities."

"Close the office for the day and volunteer for Special Olympics or Habitat for Humanity type programs. Also get your employees involved in volunteering for these activities. Not only will you be giving them the opportunity to feel good about themselves, but they will also think more of you."[23]

REALITY CHECK

"You only get out of dentistry and your community," says Howard Farran, DDS, MBA, MAGD, Phoenix, AZ, "what you put into it. Since happiness is always an inside job, I can assure you that every dentist who gets involved feels great satisfaction."[24]

45 Become a media celebrity

You've read about high-profile dentists who have achieved celebrity status on a national and even international scale. Start small. "Think globally but act locally."

FROM THE SUCCESS FILES

"Mark McMahon, DDS, made himself a media mini-celebrity in Tucson, AZ, due in part to pro bono work in his community that landed him radio and TV appearances on local stations."

McMahon established partnerships with local charities, including a homeless shelter and a shelter for battered women, and offered free dental services to their members. He also contacted local media to inquire if this "story" was of interest. As a result, several TV crews showed up, filmed him treating patients, and later aired the segments on the evening news.

"Local television news stations loved the emotional element," Dr. McMahon says. "And it was obviously rewarding for me to see patients who'd been in pain for months, talking about how glad they were to be relieved of their toothaches after we'd treated them."[25]

When Dr. Kenneth Rawlinson, DDS, Riverside, RI, first saw "Extreme Makeover" on TV, says *Dental Practice Report*, he saw a chance to have some fun, bring a little sparkle to the residents of his tiny state and boost his practice visibility.

So Dr. Rawlinson contacted cosmetic surgeon Dr. Curtis Perry and the pair pitched the idea to the state's ABC affiliate, WLNE-6. The station jumped at the chance, especially because the doctors donated their services and already had buy-in from the makeover recipients. The result was three news segments followed by a special for the grand unveiling.

The station has since signed on for additional segments and the applications are pouring in for makeovers. So far the exposure has brought in only five or six new patients. But the results far outweigh that measurement, Dr. Rawlinson says. "Most of all, it's been a blast. But we've also seen internal referrals skyrocket. It's creating a source of pride for my patients who can say, 'Hey, that's my dentist.'"[26]

---

46 Media exposure boosts credibility

"It's amazing," says Bernardine Cruz, DVM, Aliso Viejo, CA, "how your credibility goes up when you appear on local radio or TV or are written about in the local newspaper. You're the same doctor you've always been, but being in the media suddenly makes you an 'expert;' makes people think, 'You must *really* be good.' Such exposure on a regular basis is a low-cost, highly-effective way to become better known in your community and will greatly benefit your practice."

Dr. Cruz has done 1-minute segments on local radio in Los Angeles. She also does segments for "Smart Solutions," a nationally broadcast, cable HG-TV (House and Gardens) show. The following are some of her suggestions for getting exposure in your local media:

The smaller the market, the better your chances are of getting on radio, TV, or written about in the local newspaper.

Write the producer of a radio or TV show (or newspaper columnist) for which you think there is a good fit with your message. Keep it low-key such as: "If you ever need someone to talk about_____, please call me." Include a brief background about yourself and your practice. If a need arises, you may be called (which is exactly the way it worked for Dr. Cruz when she first started out).

More effective than writing is simply going to the station or newspaper, introducing yourself to the proper person, and asking the same question. (If such a person happens to be a patient of yours, it's really easy.)

Have a topic of interest, says Dr. Cruz. The interview isn't going to be about you or your practice. It's going to be about a topic of interest to their listeners, viewers, or readers—something that affects them personally.

Have realistic expectations. It may take many "tries" before you're called for an interview. When it happens, be willing to do it on short notice or, conversely, accept a last-minute cancellation (because of a late-breaking story). Your patients will be impressed but it will likely take repeated exposures in the media to attract new patients. In any event, says Dr. Cruz, it will be a "fun" experience.

47 Public service

There are countless nonprofit organizations that provide desperately needed dental care to underserved populations throughout this country.

A few hours of your time can bring years of comfort and dignity to deserving patients who fall through the cracks of most public health programs including Medicare (which doesn't offer dental benefits) and Medicaid (which limits adult dental benefits). Because of their ages or disabilities, many cannot work or afford expensive dental treatment.

Donated Dental Services (DDS) for example, is a humanitarian project of the National Foundation of Dentistry for the Handicapped (NFDH), a charitable affiliate of the American Dental Association. As a volunteer for DDS, you can provide direct service to this often overlooked and at-risk population. Designed by dentists to be as simple as possible, DDS is one of the largest dental health programs in the nation. You decide who you will treat. You don't have to leave your office. You determine your treatment plan. There's no paperwork or administrative responsibilities, and the patients are reliable and so grateful for the difference you make in their lives.

"Since the inception of Donated Dental Services," says Frank A. Maggio, DDS, NFDH chairman, "program volunteers have helped more than 55,000 disabled, elderly, medically compromised people. More than 11,500 volunteer dentists and 2700 laboratories generously have given these people over $65 million worth of comprehensive care."[27]

FROM THE SUCCESS FILES

"DDS is such a rewarding experience," says Betty A. Haberkamp, DDS, Chicago, IL. "The patients I've treated are always so appreciative of what I do. What truly makes this worthwhile are the smiles they've hidden for so long being proudly displayed. It's a good reminder of why I chose this profession."[28]

Volunteer dentists receive an etched metal plaque from their State Dental Association and State Chapter of the NFDH that "thankfully acknowledges (recipient's name) for volunteering for the Donated Dental Services Program, a humanitarian service to the disabled, elderly and medically compromised."

For further information, contact NFDH at (888) 471-6334 or www.nfdh.org

REALITY CHECK

Public service makes your brand truly meaningful by meeting the needs of others while enriching your life.

48 Hard-learned lessons about building a brand

- Your brand is not what you say you are, but what your patient thinks you are.
- The power behind a brand name that patients insist on is undeniable. And it all begins with a promise: a promise to deliver a level of quality and service. If all goes well, it becomes a set of expectations. As those expectations are fulfilled again and again, a reputation develops.
- Branding results from a patient's overall experience with your office starting with the first moment they hear or read about your office. It's an outgrowth of the culture of your practice; the core values, the perceived quality of care, and the impression made by your staff.
- "When affection for you is the only thing that separates you or your brand from the competition in the mind of the consumer," says British author/consultant Guy Browning, "you better make damn sure that you keep in contact, that you say the right things and that you listen for any minute changes in wants, needs or expectations."[29]
- Brands take time to develop. You can't rush the process with rampant self-promotion.
- The members of your dental team are *brand ambassadors* for your practice.
- It should be the top priority of every staff member to build, protect, and represent your brand to the best of their ability.
- Brands demand consistency. "If your receptionist is rude," say consultants Olivia and Kerry Straine, "if your office manager is unhelpful when a patient needs financing, if your policies are always changing, the negative impact on your brand can destroy the clinical standards of excellence you have worked so hard to achieve."[30]
- If your brand includes "excellence," make sure that's reflected in the quality of everything about your office. Otherwise, you're sending mixed messages.
- Branding always works. It either attracts patients or it drives them away. There's no middle ground.

"Building a strong brand relationship with your customers," says Shelly Lazarus, chairman and CEO of Ogilvy & Mather Worldwide, "is not an easy challenge. It requires focus, diligence, and integrity. But the rewards are enormous. Customer loyalty is almost priceless in today's world, and only strong brands with strong brand relationships can command it."[31]

Your brand, like that of a consumer product, is based on *perception*. It's what other people think of you and your practice. To get a handle on what those perceptions are, use the market research ideas in Chapter 10. Patient satisfaction surveys, focus groups, "no-holds barred" staff meetings, and postappointment telephone interviews will provide valuable feedback about how others see you.

A strong practice brand also creates high levels of employee pride and is a magnet for recruiting the best employees and retaining them over time.

ACTION STEP

Schedule a staff meeting to discuss what you'd like patients to think about your practice. What aspects of your practice would you like patients to particularly notice and tell others about? Be specific and descriptive. It will put everyone in your practice on the same page.

Notes

1. When Two or Three or Four Names are Better Than One. *Hotels,* April 2004, 20.
2. Eliscu AT. How Branding Can Position Your Practice for Success. *Physician's Marketing & Management,* September 1997, 118-119.
3. Peters T. The Brand Called You. *Fast Company,* August/September, 1997.
4. Collins JC, Porras JI. *Built to Last: Successful Habits of Visionary Companies,* HarperBusiness, 1997.
5. Moser M. United We Brand. Boston: *Harvard Business School Press,* 2003.
6. Schwab D. What Your Staff Needs to Know About Marketing Your Practice. *Dental Economics,* January 1999, 50-53, 95.
7. Rosenthal L. A Top 10 List of Mistakes in Practice Management. *Dental Economics,* April 1998.
8. Wilde JA. Regrets? I've Got a Few. *Dental Economics,* May 2003, 124-128.
9. Bonner P. Elements of a Successful Aesthetic Dental Practice. *Dentistry Today,* April, 1998, 50-57.
10. Aaker DA. Building Strong Brands. New York: *Free Press,* 1996.
11. McNally D, Speak KD. *Be Your Own Brand.* San Francisco: Berrett-Koehler Publishers, Inc, 2002.
12. On Target. Full Speed Ahead. Target Corporation Annual Report, 2003.
13. Dallin JB. Why Have a Web Site? Part 1. *Dental Economics,* January 2003, 96.
14. Dorfman W. Go Hollywood, *Dental Economics,* May, 2003, 124-128.
15. Moser M. *United We Brand,* Boston, MA: Harvard Business School Press, 2003.

16. Gobé M. *Emotional Branding*, New York: Allworth Press, 2001.
17. Roberts P. The Agenda—Total Teamwork. *Fast Company*, April 1999, p 48.
18. Trost L. Editor's Note: Matters of the Heart. *Woman Dentist Journal*, February 2004, 6.
19. Fombrun CJ, Riel CV. *Fame & Fortune*. Upper Saddle River, NJ: Financial Times/Prentice-Hall, 2003.
20. Nash RW. Building the Esthetic Practice. *Dental Practice Report*, June 2002, 30-36.
21. http://www.wowseminars.com.
22. Yankelovich Monitor® April 15, 2004.
23. Schwartz S. Effectively Marketing Your Practice. *Dental Economics*, November 2003, 68-74.
24. Farran H. Charitable Dentistry, Missionary Dentistry, & The Spiritual Side of Dentistry. *Dental Town Magazine*, February 2004, 10.
25. Yoder SV. Make It Mean Something. *Successful Meetings*, February 2004, 27-28.
26. Makeover Shows Whet Public's Esthetic Appetite. *Dental Practice Report*, March 2004, 10, 12.
27. National Foundation of Dentistry for the Handicapped. 2002-2003 Annual Report Denver, CO: NFDH.
28. *Special Smiles*, Illinois Foundation of Dentistry for the Handicapped.
29. Browning G. *Innervation: Rewire Yourself for the New Economy*. New York: Perseus Publishing, 2003.
30. Straine OM, Straine KK. Success Simply Isn't Enough . . . You Can Experience Significance! *Dentistry Today*, September 2003, 118-121.
31. Lazarus SD. What it Takes to Become Valued to Customers. *Pfizer Annual Report*, 2001, 7.

4

Long-Range Strategic Planning

Strategic planning is the fundamental process by which an organization determines specific action steps to achieve future goals. It is the map that guides your activities on the way to your destination by identifying what needs to be done, by whom, with what resources, and by what date. Planning allows the organization as a whole to focus on the right priorities and activities to accomplish its goals and is one of the key management activities that will allow an organization to proactively manage its growth.

Strategic planning starts with figuring out where you and your practice are at the moment, where you're headed, where you'll be a year or two from now, and how you'll get there. Will the focus be the same? How about the priorities? Will you be serving the same patient base or entirely different segments of the population? Will you continue to offer the same mix of services or shift gears?

Your answers to such questions will influence everything in your practice starting with *what* you do and *how* you do it: the kinds of patients you attract, your standards for quality and service, the location of your office, your fees, equipment, continuing education, whom you hire; the size of your staff, how you promote the practice, the pace of the practice, the overhead, and on and on.

REALITY CHECK

There's no "correct" answer as such. No one size that fits all. What's best for *you* will depend on your values, philosophy of practice, priorities, and answers to the many questions posed throughout this book.

49 Conduct a S.W.O.T. analysis

A *S.W.O.T.* analysis is an important component of long-range strategic planning that is widely used in industry. It's an acronym for: Strengths, Weaknesses, Opportunities, and Threats. A critical assessment of these issues is essential to develop an action plan for the future growth of your practice.

Strengths. Strengths refer to the things you and your staff do exceptionally well, perhaps better than anyone else. Or this strength may be something about your practice that gives it a competitive advantage, such as your location, high-tech equipment, unique services, office hours, caliber of personnel, or any of a host of other things. You need to know what these strengths are and make sure you maintain them.

To help identify your strengths, discuss with your staff such questions as the following:

- What has made our practice successful?
- Why do patients bypass other practices, especially those with lower fees, to come to us?
- For what are we best known?
- Why do physicians and other professional people refer patients to our office?
- What accounts for patient loyalty?
- What are we most proud of?

Weaknesses. Weaknesses refer to anything that has an adverse effect on productivity, profitability, patient satisfaction, staff morale, reputation, and practice growth. These may include the following:

- Things you're doing that you *shouldn't* be doing, such as long waits in the office, high-pressure tactics when presenting treatment plans, overbooking and then rushing patients and, perhaps most important, cutting corners to improve profitability.
- Things you need to do *more* of, such as continuing education, delegation, staff meetings, patient education, networking with physicians, and market research.
- Aspects of your practice that you may have let slip such as preventive care and your re-care system, staff training, addition of new equipment, and office décor.

How does this happen?

Part of the problem may be that you're *too busy*, which at first may seem like a good problem to have. But the question is: Are you busier than you "should be?" Has an ever-increasing schedule begun to affect the quality of patient care, patient acceptance of treatment plans, staff relations, or perhaps your health and disposition? If so, you may be caught up in what I call the "runaway practice."

The runaway practice is bolstered by word-of-mouth referrals, networking, increased visibility in your community, perhaps by managed care. That's the good news. The bad news is that sooner or later it reaches the point of diminishing returns, at which point deteriorating service, patient care, and staff morale (not to mention your own health and disposition) begin to have a *negative impact* on patient satisfaction and practice growth.

If it's happened in your practice, there are several options:

1. Hire an associate to lighten your workload.
2. Hire additional clinical or office personnel.
3. Consider cutting back on procedures you no longer want to do (see Secrets #193 and #194).
4. Continue at the current pace, but keep in mind the law of diminishing returns.
5. Consider dropping low-paying managed care plans or perhaps opting completely out of managed care (see Chapter 5).

FROM THE SUCCESS FILES

"I have focused my practice solely on aesthetic dentistry," says Christopher Pescatore, DMD, Danville, CA. "I no longer have to run from room to room to see patients. I can spend more time with each patient and build valuable relationships, something I could never do in a large practice setting. A typical day for me is seeing anywhere from one to six patients, depending on the procedures I'm performing. I usually work a four-day week from 8:30 a.m. to 4:45 p.m. with a one hour lunch break. The bottom line: I work less, make more money, spend more time with my family, and consider my patients friends. What more could I ask for?"[1]

HARD-LEARNED LESSONS

"New patients are essential," says world-renowned clinician Peter E. Dawson, DDS, St. Petersburg, FL, "but trying to treat too many patients is counterproductive and unfair to patients. Too many patients is also the most common obstacle to clinical excellence, which is the single most important factor that determines how successful a practice becomes."[2]

"Our profession seems fixated on trying to see more patients," says Ron Schefdore, DMD, Burr Ridge, IL, "even discounting fees until we end up working for insurance companies. We churn out 20, 30, 40 patients a day, or more. The dentist, staff and equipment take a beating every day."[3]

"Being busy isn't a badge of honor," says Leonard J. Press, OD, FAAO, FCVD, Fair Lawn, NJ. "It's a badge of stupidity."

Opportunities. Opportunities refer to what you and your staff could be doing (that you're not now doing) that would produce increased profitability and/or practice growth. Opportunities also include things that if done *differently* (than you're now doing) would achieve better results. Consider, for example, the following matrix representing four possibilities:

	Current Services	New Services
Current Patients	1	2
New Patients	3	4

The easiest of the four is number 1: getting more of your current patients to use more of your current services. It requires nothing new except improved communication skills.

The hardest of the four is number 4: acquiring new patients for new services. In this case, you need to acquire both expertise and new patients.

Chapters 5 and 6 will include the action steps needed to mine some of these opportunities.

Threats. Threats refer to any issue that may prevent you and your staff from reaching the goals you've set for your practice. To help identify these issues, consider such questions as the following:

- What socioeconomic or demographic shifts are occurring in the community that have (or will have) an impact on your practice?
- What are the greatest challenges facing your practice over the next few years that must be overcome to ensure your continued success?

- What would happen if you reduced your dependence on dental insurance or perhaps eliminated it completely?
- What is the "competition" doing in terms of: services offered; equipment; hours of operation; professional fees; participation in third-party plans, advertising?

REALITY CHECK

Recently, I visited a dentist in the southeast who told me about a relatively new practice about 2 miles away that was "clobbering" his well-regarded but aging practice, and to which a sizeable number of his patients had transferred.

"Have you ever visited that office?" I inquired.

"No, I haven't," he admitted.

I convinced him that a visit to that office was in order. In fact it was a *must*. We called, asked if we could come by, and were enthusiastically invited to do so later that afternoon.

The contrast between the two offices was immediately obvious. The layout of this office, the artwork, color scheme, lighting, fresh flowers, the soft music wafting through the office, the multiple treatment room computer systems with integrated clinical software, the digital X-ray and practice management software, and the friendliness of everyone were *spectacular*!

When we left a while later, the dentist who accompanied me confided, "I now know what my problem is."

In the words of educator John Dewey, a problem well-stated is half-solved.

---

50 Hard-learned lessons about long-range strategic planning

Long-range planning is the key to turning the dreams for your practice into reality. It provides the mechanism to coordinate and focus the activities of day-to-day practice. It identifies the most important priorities and ensures that everyone is rowing in the same direction.

There is no magic formula for strategic planning. If you were to ask ten management consultants, you'd probably get ten different methods, all variations on the same theme. The truth is that planning is not an exact science and the technique is less important than the process itself.

Make sure that staff members are involved in the S.W.O.T. analysis. Called *participative management*, this group effort fosters commitment, team spirit, and practice growth.

Strategic planning is not a result or an outcome but rather an ongoing process. Gary Hamel, a leading strategy consultant, says, "Strategizing is not a once-a-year rain dance, nor is it a once-a-decade consulting project. To be useful, it must become part of the bedrock of the company."[4]

Notes

1. Pescatore C. The Wonderful World of Adhesive Dentistry. *Dental Economics,* July 2003, 46-50, 122.
2. Dawson PE. Want a Thriving Practice? Concentrate on Clinical Excellence. *Dental Economics,* October 1992, 78-79.
3. Schefdore R. Better Service, Better Dentistry, Better Income. *Dentistry Today,* December 2003, 10.
4. Hamel G. Killer Strategies That Make Shareholders Rich. *Fortune,* June 23, 1997, 80.

5

Golden Opportunities for Practice Growth

This chapter is an outgrowth of the S.W.O.T. analysis described in Chapter 4.

51 Acres of diamonds

Do you recall the parable "Acres of Diamonds" about an ambitious farmer in ancient Persia who was always looking for new opportunities? One day, he heard about the tremendous wealth that diamonds could bring him and that they were being found in great numbers in far away lands. Believing a great fortune was within his grasp, the farmer sold his land and embarked on a long search.

He journeyed throughout Europe and the Middle East but without success. Finally, discouraged and penniless, he threw himself into the violent waters between the Pillars of Hercules, destroying himself and all his dreams.

Meanwhile, the man who purchased the farmer's land was walking his camel by a stream that cut through his newly purchased property. When the camel stopped to drink from the stream, a bright sparkle caught the new owner's eye. It was a diamond.

If the farmer had carefully examined his own property, he would have fulfilled his wildest dreams. It was harboring literally *acres of diamonds* although they were not visible to the untrained eye.

Later this farm was developed into the famous diamond mines of Golconda.

This parable was retold to over 6000 audiences in the late 1800s by Russell H. Conwell, the founder and first president of Temple University. It illustrates the importance of looking in your "own backyard" for the things you seek in life.

Here are some "backyard" opportunities for practice growth.

52 The largest influx of patients in history

"We've been asleep at the switch not to recognize the growing need for dentists to care for the largest influx of patients in history," says Peter Dawson, DDS, founder of the Dawson Center for Advanced Dental Study in St. Petersburg, FL. "The 'over-50' market is huge and growing, and their needs are great because they still have their teeth. They also have periodontal disease, excessive wear problems, cracked teeth, and a ton of deteriorating amalgams, and most of all of them want good-looking smiles."[1]

On the same note, Jimmy Eubank, DDS, director of the postgraduate Esthetics Continuum at Louisiana State University School of Dentistry, had this to say: "I believe the public is a sleeping giant of demand because they really don't know what dentistry can do for them. But when they learn, there is going to be an exponentially increasing demand for the dentist who can truly deliver excellence in aesthetics and occlusion."

"The best days of dentistry, the 'golden days of dentistry,'" he adds, "are still ahead. The profession is on the threshold of an unbelievable demand for its services."[2]

53 Follow-up patients who "want to think about" recommended treatment

"How many patients in your file cabinet have outstanding restorative work that needs to be completed?" asks speaker/coach Janet Hagerman, RDH. "Would your money be better spent marketing for new patients or treating the restorative needs of patients who already exist in your practice and who already have a (presumably good) relationship with you?"[3]

HARD-LEARNED LESSON
Waiting for patients to take the initiative about recommended treatment that they "want to think about" about is wishful thinking.

FROM THE SUCCESS FILES
"In many instances," says Samuel M. Strong, DDS, Little Rock, AR, "the patient wants to have implant treatment performed, but is simply not ready to do it because of financial concerns, time, occupational restraints, or personal matters unknown to you and your staff."

"Follow up with prospective patients," Dr. Strong suggests, "for some period of time (6 to 12 months or more) to maintain the relationship. Just reminding the patient through letters, brochures, or other printed material of the benefits of implant therapy can improve the chances that they return to your office when they are ready to proceed. We have seen patients wait two years or more before returning to review their options—and then decide to continue on with the proposed treatment."[4]

54 Status update exams

"When I audit records in dental practices," says consultant/speaker Annette Ashley Linder, BS, RDH, "I find that most patients received a new patient exam when they first entered the practice but in many cases, not since. Because of time constraints at the routine dental hygiene (recall) appointment, we tend to keep the patient in the system with a periodic oral exam that does not allow enough time to establish a meaningful dialogue with the patient."

"It's amazing," Ms. Linder says, "the amount of dentistry that is detected, presented and accepted when there is ample time allotted for a comprehensive, bring-things-up-to-date status exam. Whenever we have an opening in the hygiene schedule (cancellation, failed appointment, or unbooked appointment) the time is efficiently utilized to give the patient in the chair an updated status exam. Extending time with the patient in the chair allows the hygienist to update the radiographs, complete the periodontal examination, tour the mouth with the intra-oral camera, display patient-education modules, discuss treatment options, and answer any patient questions."

"As a result, what would have been unproductive time is now an opportunity to schedule more treatment and increase practice profitability."[5]

ACTION STEP

"It may be time," adds consultant/speaker Debra Engelhardt-Nash, "to look at patients who have been in your practice for 5 years or longer as though they were new to your practice and you are seeing them for the first time: more objectively, more comprehensively, more focused. An increase in treatment acceptance from patients of record is certain."[6]

---

55 The sleeping giant in every dental practice

"I consider inactive patients to be the sleeping giant in every dental practice," says consultant/speaker Linda Miles, CSP, CMC, "by which I mean there is literally a goldmine in most dental office filing systems comprised of files of once active patients. These are individuals who have not been to see the dentist for a year or more."

"Once they're contacted," Ms. Miles adds, "large percentages of these patients rekindle their relationship with the practice translating into thousands of dollars to the bottom line."[7]

Letters and postcards will reactivate some of these patients, but not many. Most patients receiving these mailings agree with the need to return, put them in the pile of "things to do," and promptly forget about them. Blame it on inertia.

ACTION STEP

The most effective way to reactivate such patients is to *make it easy* for them to make an appointment. Here's how.

Start with 25 randomly selected patients who have not been in the practice for a year or more. Have a knowledgeable, well-trained staff member *telephone* these patients. Let them know how long it's been since they were last seen by the hygienist and/or doctor and inquire if they would like to make an appointment.

The staff member may learn the patient has moved away or possibly switched to another dentist. Or the patient may say, "I'm doing fine and don't care to make an appointment."

Let's just focus on the easy-to-activate patients who say:

"Has it really been that long?"
"I know it's been a long time. I've been meaning to call you."
"I've been waiting for you to call me."

You'll hear these replies far more often than you might guess, any of which will lead to an appointment.

Needless to say, only a handful of favorable responses more than warrants telephoning the balance of your inactive patients.

HARD-LEARNED LESSON

Think of these as "courtesy calls," not "sales calls." Being pushy when patients show no interest in making an appointment will surely backfire and cause resentment.

56 Tap unused employee health benefits

Many employer-based health benefit packages provide dental care benefits that must be used in the course of a calendar year.

FROM THE SUCCESS FILES

"In late October or early November, we start running reports from our dental software to get a list of patients with treatment plans in the current year that never scheduled an opportunity to have the work done," says Howard Farran, DDS, MBA, MAGD, Phoenix, AZ. "My front office staff cross references the names on this report with the patients' charts to verify what insurance benefits they have used so far. We then send a letter to patients who have unused benefits left to cover the work, or a portion of the work that has been treatment planned for them. By sending the letter, we are informing our patients of their remaining dental benefits, as well as giving them a reminder about the treatment they should complete before their dental concern gets worse."[8]

REALITY CHECK
Many patients simply forget to use health plan benefits during the course of the year. As a result, they enter into the final months of each year with benefits they must essentially use or lose. You can do your patients a great service by reminding them to take advantage of any unused health plan benefits before year's end—*and* have a busier-than-usual December.

57 E-mail communication

"An effective e-mail program gives your office a high-tech image," says Ralph Laurie, President, CAESY Education Systems. "Think of the possibilities that e-mail opens up: appointment reminders, welcome letters, birthday greetings, recall notices, patient newsletters, post-op check in, and patient-education presentations."

"The beauty of e-mail," Mr. Laurie says, "is that it is still in the romance stage. People like to send and receive e-mail. There's an excitement when you hear the chime and the voice announcing, 'You've got mail.' E-mail is a welcomed, personal method of communication that strengthens the doctor-patient relationship."

"Begin gathering your patients' e-mail addresses during the check-in process," Mr. Laurie recommends. "It may take several months, but you will soon have a comprehensive e-mail list with which you can begin to communicate with patients, quickly and cost-effectively."[9]

FROM THE SUCCESS FILES

Corine Leech, office manager for Thomas K. Hedge, DDS, West Chester, OH, recalls, "When we started asking patients if we can get their e-mail addresses, they asked why. We told them we'd like to e-mail them a newsletter, information and appointment reminders. They said, 'Great!' Since then, they've been asking, 'Hey, where's that newsletter that we should be receiving?' I'm really surprised at how many people prefer that means of communication."[10]

REALITY CHECK

According to a 2003 Harris Interactive survey, 67 percent of adults (140 million people) are now online, which strongly suggests that it is worthwhile to target an e-mail audience. A January 2001 survey noted that 81 percent of the online population wished to receive e-mail reminders for preventive care while 83 percent of them wanted follow-up e-mails after visits to doctors. Considering the trend of e-mail growth, Internet access will surely become the standard as the preferred patient contact medium.[11]

HARD-LEARNED LESSON

"In any e-mail newsletter you send," says Chris Kammer, DDS, Madison, WI, "always make sure to include a clickable link that will send people directly to your Web site so they can learn more about your practice. A note of caution: always give your e-mail recipients a chance to unsubscribe to your e-newsletter so you can avoid potential issues that may arise from unwanted e-mails."[12]

58 Expand your service base

An increase in production will occur if more services are added to the dental menu.

"Here's an example," says Richard Miller, DDS, Alexandria, VA. "Is your soft-tissue management program state-of-the-art? Do you perform the latest diagnostic techniques? How often do you probe? Do you use the latest irrigation materials? Are fluoride treatments a part of your hygiene program? What about a laser to treat non-healed periodontal sites? How often do your patients have maintenance visits?"[13]

"There are so many great endodontic systems out there today that have made endo faster, easier and better than ever," says Louis Malcmacher, DDS, Cleveland Heights, OH. "There is no reason every general practitioner should not be doing anterior endodontics at the very least. The better and more proficient you become in endodontics, especially the *diagnosis* of teeth that need endodontics, the busier you'll be and the busier your endodontist will be."[14]

"One hour whitening," Dr. Malcmacher says, "has attracted more patients to the office than anything I can remember in recent history. This is something patients want, something they see in magazines and on television, something they will pay for, and it's a service you can provide easily."

"Porcelain veneers are (another) underutilized service that has great potential to grow the aesthetic part of your practice."

ACTION STEP

"Choose those services that interest you," advises Dr. Malcmacher, "and those which you are comfortable providing for your patients. No matter which new procedures you choose to add to your menu of dental services, these line extensions help expand the service base to your patients, provide an opportunity to grow your practice, and provide patients with the ability to get the newest treatments dentistry has to offer from the person they trust most—you, their family dentist."

---

59 Drop low-paying managed care plans

"Never join or participate in any managed care plan," says consultant/speaker Tom Limoli, Jr., "that reduces your usual fee, *unless* you need additional patients to fill empty chairs."[15]

FROM THE SUCCESS FILES

"My practice is located on the south side of Chicago," says Lou Graham, DDS, "in a community known as Hyde Park, which houses the University of Chicago. Over 10 years ago, the university started offering a very cheap HMO to its employees as an alternative to expensive private insurance, and off went hundreds of my patients! Humbling to say, our monthly income was dramatically affected, but I would not submit my care to such low fees and low expectations. I think what truly hurt was that I thought my patients would see the 'value' in my care, but for those who left, I guess I was wrong."

"Within three years, most of those patients returned, many with work that was never done, worsened periodontal conditions, and poor relationships with their new dentists. I realized then that they now understood the value of my high standards of care."[16]

"After joining a handful of plans in our area," says orthodontist Tom Barron, DDS, MS, Towson, MD, "it became apparent that we were working harder, employing more people, generating more gross revenue—but not necessarily taking home more money."

"After several years, we started to gradually discontinue our relationship with these plans. More than 18 months later, we are noticeably less busy. Scheduling problems have begun to ease and the stress levels have decreased considerably. The entire staff can spend more time with patients and day-to-day operations are generally smoother. Much to our surprise, there has not been an economic downtown in the practice as we had anticipated. Gross income has actually increased slightly, and the net has improved. In other words, we are less busy and making more money."[17]

REALITY CHECK

"Dental benefit plans are in the world to stay," says consultant/speaker James R. Pride, DDS. "For some dentists they will remain important aspects of their practice. Yet, there is nothing that says you have to participate in them if you feel you are not benefiting as a result. If you do decide to reduce participation in such plans, do so slowly and be prepared for some patients to leave. However, if your practice is operating with the proper systems and staff training, it's likely you'll experience little or no patient loss. Research shows that of those patients who do choose to leave, some will return to a quality practice after experiencing dentistry elsewhere after approximately 12 months. These patients recognize the value of the experience provided in these outstanding practices and are willing to pay for that experience."[18]

ACTION STEP

"Take things one step at a time," advises consultant Bill Rossi. "Drop one PPO at a time. Most importantly, have concrete plans to strengthen the remainder of your practice to compensate for any patient attrition. In short, have a plan."[19]

60 Attract more fee-for-service patients

"As some experts note, dentists who want to recruit and retain more full-fee paying patients, must meet an emerging 'gold standard' of service," say Bob Kehoe and Dan Blunk, editor and associate editor of *Dental Practice & Finance*. "These sources contend that dental teams must be exceptionally attentive to meeting patients' needs, desires, and expectations. Greater attention also must be paid to patients' comfort, schedules and preferences."[20]

"Some dentists ply their patients with gourmet coffee, 10 varieties of tea, freshly baked cookies and a docking station for their laptops," says *Dental Practice Report*. "Still other dental offices are wooing harried patients with massages, hot wax hand baths and warm moist towels like you get in sushi houses."[21]

REALITY CHECK

"Many businesses believe packing their offerings with what they consider to be 'value-added services' will attract customers," say consultants Fred Crawford and Ryan Mathews. "It explains why coffee bars can be found in bookstores. The problem is that for most consumers, these services really take a back seat to some very basic competencies that many businesses have failed to master. Consumers make it clear they are looking for fewer gimmicks and more delivery when it comes to service. If the service provided at the moment of interaction is deficient, all the value-added services in the world aren't going to help the business hang on to that customer. This suggests that businesses seeking to dominate on service would do better taking the money they have been putting into all those extra services and put it into employee screening, training, measuring and rewarding in an effort to provide point-of-interaction value to the customer."[22]

Hard-Learned Lesson

"The culture of Southwest Airlines," says Jeffrey A. Krames in *What the Best CEOs Know: 7 Exceptional Leaders and Their Lessons for Transforming Any Business*, "is probably its major competitive advantage. The intangibles are more important than the tangibles because you can always imitate the tangibles. You can buy the airplane, you can rent the ticket counter space. But the hardest thing for someone to emulate is the spirit of your people."[23]

61 Hard-learned lessons about attracting fee-for-service patients

"In order to attract fee-for-service patients," says Russell G. Rosenquist, DDS, Glenview, IL, past president of the American Academy of Dental Practice Administration, you must take the following steps:

- Have high-level clinical competency and an office that runs smoothly and efficiently.
- Have a physical facility that is convenient, modern, and noticeably clean (not just clean, but *noticeably* clean).
- Have a team that is outgoing, well-groomed, dressed professionally, have great smiles, love people, and are well-trained for their respective jobs. In addition, the respect between the doctor and staff must be obvious.
- Have a local study club with whom you can talk about practice-related problems and share confidences.
- Build the patient's confidence and trust in you. *Earned trust* is the key to patient acceptance and loyalty.
- Give patients an easy-to-understand reason to return for periodic maintenance visits and then pre-appoint them. Over 90% will comply.
- Don't be afraid to ask for referrals. The phrase with which I'm comfortable, Dr. Rosenquist says, is, "We need and appreciate your referral of friends to our office." Start saying that to patients and you may be surprised to have them reply, "I didn't realize you were taking new patients."

62 Networking

Networking with physicians and related healthcare practitioners has tremendous potential for getting new patients into your practice on a recurring basis. Because of its importance, Chapter 6 is devoted to this topic.

Notes

1. Blaes J. Interviewing a Giant of Dentistry. *Dental Economics,* January 2004, 66-70.
2. Bonner P. Integrating Cosmetic Dentistry into the General Dental Practice. *Dentistry Today,* April 1999, 46-51.
3. Hagerman J. Boring Basics: The Magic Potion for Success. *Dentistry Today,* October 2003, 80-85.
4. Strong SM. Nine Steps to Profitability with Implant Prosthetics. *Dental Economics,* May 2003, 100-106.
5. Linder AA. Hygiene Up Close. *Dental Economics,* January 2003, 46-52.
6. Nash DE. Building the Esthetic Practice Through Recall. *Dental Practice Report,* June 2000, 10-14.
7. Miles L. Dynamic Dentistry. Virginia Beach, VA: *Link Publishing,* 2003.
8. Farran H. The Importance of Our Today's Dental Unused Benefits Letter. *DentalTown Magazine,* November 2003, 4.
9. Laurie R. Don't Let Your Web Site Be a Disappointment. *Dental Economics,* January 2000, 48-50.
10. Make Your Web Site Reach Out to Patients, *Dental Economics,* August 2000, 38-40, 170.
11. Guiliana J, Homisak L, Levin RS et al. How-To Insights for Expanding Your Practice. *Podiatry Today,* December 2003, 54-58.
12. Kammer C. The Future of Advertising: E-mail Marketing. *Dental Angle Online Magazine,* Fall 2001.
13. Miller R. Recession-Proof Your Practice. *Dentistry Today,* March 2002, 96-101.
14. Malcmacher L. Line Extensions. *Dental Economics,* April 2004, 68.
15. Limoli T. Jr. What Write-Off? *Dental Economics,* August 2002, 28.
16. Graham L. Base Your Treatment Plan on Saving Enamel! *Dental Economics,* December, 2003, 84-86, 111.
17. Barron T. What's Your Next Move? *Dental Economics,* April 2003, 76-82, 149.
18. Taking Your Practice to a New Level. St. Paul, MN: *3M Dental Products,* 1999.
19. Rossi B. Cutting Out the PPOs. *Dental Economics,* March 2001, 68-78.
20. Kehoe B, Blunk D. The New 'Gold Standard' in Patient Service. *Dental Practice & Finance,* February 1998, 15-19.
21. Kehoe B, Blunk D. Office Amenities. *Dental Practice Report,* March 2001, 14.
22. Crawford F, Mathews R. *The Myth of Excellence.* New York: Crown Business, 2001.
23. Krames JA. *What the Best CEOs Know: 7 Exceptional Leaders and Their Lessons for Transforming Any Business.* New York: McGraw-Hill, 2003.

6

Secrets of Savvy Networking

"What's the worst thing you can say about another doctor?" asks otolargyngologist/allergist Martin H. Zwerling of Aiken, SC. "That he's incompetent, lazy, dishonest? No, the worst thing you can say is, 'I never heard of him.' Building your own practice," he adds, "means developing effective relationships with your colleagues in the community."[1]

Networking is one means of getting known and developing mutually beneficial relationships with colleagues and other healthcare practitioners that lead to an exchange of information and often, reciprocal referrals. These include dental specialists; general dentists (if you're a specialist); primary care physicians; pediatricians; cosmetic surgeons; ear, nose, and throat physicians (ENTs); orthopedic surgeons; pharmacists; hospital emergency rooms; among others.

63 Dental specialists

"I have found that very few specialists are aware of what's possible with aesthetic dentistry," says Stephen D. Poss, DDS, Smyrna, TN. "I visited the area's dental specialists: orthodontists, periodontists, oral surgeons, and endodontists, and took them to lunch. Over lunch I showed them pictures and discussed the latest things we were doing in cosmetic dentistry. The goal was to make them aware of our services and of the great strides that have been made in aesthetic dentistry.

It took a significant amount of time and effort, but it has had an enormous impact on my practice."[2]

64 ENTS and orthopedic surgeons

"ENT and orthopedic surgeons are important sources of temporomandibular disorder (TMD) patients," says periodontist Michael E. Kossak, DDS, Washington, DC. "Patients frequently see them for symptoms that include TMD, but they are not equipped to handle this problem and welcome the opportunity to refer these patients to someone they trust. Patients seek treatment from the ENT specialist for such symptoms as earache, tinnitus, blocked eustachian tubes, etc. When there is no pathologic reason for the symptoms other than TMD, referral to a dentist is frequently made. Patients from orthopedic surgeons usually complain about headaches, vague neck and shoulder pain, or whiplash."[3]

65 Cosmetic surgeons

How do you get patients from a plastic surgeon?" asks William M. Dorfman, DDS, Beverly Hills, CA. "The surgeon is not interested in sending you patients, at least not at first," he says. "However, the surgeon is highly interested in getting patients from you."

"What you can do," suggests Dr. Dorfman, "is call or write and say for example, 'Because I do cosmetic dentistry, my patients sometimes ask me about cosmetic surgery and who I'd recommend. I'd like to have someone to refer them to. Why don't we have lunch and talk about this? And would you bring some of your practice brochures?' Unless the plastic surgeon is booked solid for the year, you will eventually have lunch or at least a conversation. Another approach," says Dr. Dorfman, "is to call and ask if you can observe surgery. That way you can see not only what goes on in the plastic surgeon's practice, but establish a personal relationship as well."[4]

FROM THE SUCCESS FILES

"I sent a letter to all of the plastic surgeons in Cincinnati," says Tom Hedge, DDS, Cincinnati, OH, "that outlined my interest in learning what they could offer my patients. Five out of 20 responded and I met with each one. I recommend meeting plastic surgeons at their offices. It gives you an opportunity to see their albums of 'before and after' cases and to see first hand where you will send your patients."[5]

Scott Coleman, DDS, FAGD, Houston, TX, whose special interest is cosmetic dentistry, asked a cosmetic surgeon he knew socially whether his chapter of the American Academy of Cosmetic Surgery would be interested in a talk on the subject of "How Dentistry Can Improve a Person's Appearance." The answer was "yes." Dr. Coleman's presentation was well-received and led in turn to a network of cosmetic surgeons from whom he receives frequent referrals and to whom he is able to refer patients expressing an interest in cosmetic surgery.

66 Cardiologists

"Communication between dentists and physicians is critical in the proper diagnosis and treatment of all diseases," reports *Dentistry Today,* "especially heart disease, since the longer it goes untreated, the greater the risk of heart attack."[6]

"I've helped patients with heart conditions," says Academy of General Dentistry (AGD) spokesman E. Mac Edington, DDS, MAGD, ABGD, "by diagnosing dental problems that were causing local infections. By eliminating a local infection involving a tooth or the gums, patients have been able to decrease blood pressure medications and improve overall health."[6]

67 Neurologists, ENTs, and internists

"The alarming rate of undiagnosed cases of occlusal disease and the willingness of patients to accept occlusal therapy treatment," says author Jerry Simon, DDS, "creates an enormous opportunity for dentists to expand their practices, provide better treatment, and increase annual gross revenues by at least 10 to 20 percent."

"It's important to realize," Dr. Simon says, "that a majority of patients who suffer from pain due to malocclusion are in the care of medical doctors who have not been trained to recognize bite problems and therefore are unable to successfully treat them. To facilitate referrals, dentists should get into contact with neurologists, ENTs, and internists in their community and educate them about the importance of proper occlusion."[7]

68 Pediatricians

The American Academy of Pediatric Dentistry Foundation's public education campaign on children's oral health is called *Good Health Starts Here*. It targets caregivers, adolescents, and other healthcare professionals who serve children. Among the campaign materials are colorful posters and brochures intended for expecting mothers and primary caregivers of children up to the age of six. They illustrate the integral connection between oral health and overall health and provide guidelines on how to care for children's teeth during infancy and early childhood. The four areas of concentration are oral hygiene, diet and nutrition, dental visits, and fluoride.

ACTION STEP

These materials can be purchased for display in your office and/or local pediatricians' offices by going to www.aapd.org and clicking the "Online Store" link.

FROM THE SUCCESS FILES

Thirty percent of new patients at the offices of pediatric dentists Lee Weinstein, DMD, and Simon Cheirif, DDS, in Roslyn Heights and

Merrick, Long Island, NY, have been referred by pediatricians. Among the reasons is effective networking.

Dr. Weinstein is attending pediatric dentist at Long Island Jewish Medical Center, Schneider's Children Hospital. Dr. Cheirif is chairman of the Pediatric Dental Department at Jamaica Hospital. In networking terms, such affiliations give Drs. Weinstein and Cheirif important visibility and opportunities to lecture to hospital residents, physicians, pediatricians, and nurses, all of whom are potential referral sources.

Such lectures take place at the hospitals or, on occasion, at the physicians' private practices where staff members can also attend. Topics range from "What's new in pediatric dentistry?" to the consequences of an abscessed tooth, traumatic injury, nursing-bottle mouth, eruption hematoma, and the risk of malpractice if these conditions are neglected. "What's made these programs so effective," says Dr. Weinstein, "is the emphasis we put on the audience's needs and interests—not ours for recognition and referrals."

Laura Giannitelli, office manager for Drs. Weinstein and Cheirif, also visits local pediatricians four to six times a year to accomplish the following goals:

- Alert pediatricians and their staffs to Drs. Weinstein and Chierif's availability in the event one of their patients has a dental emergency.
- Offer literature (for patients) about such topics as dental sealants, nursing-bottle mouth, thumb sucking, dental-emergency procedures for parents, and the importance of primary teeth. One well-received giveaway has been a small supply of disposable mouth mirrors for physicians who express an interest in using them during their examination of children.
- Occasionally, Ms. Giannitelli will just bring doughnuts and coffee for everyone and make it a quick, social visit.

Such efforts help pediatricians and their staffs remember Drs. Weinstein and Cheirif when parents ask (as they invariably do) "Can you recommend a dentist for my child?"

What's worked for Drs. Weinstein and Cheirif to make their networking so effective are hospital affiliations, providing information that is relevant and helpful to the people with whom they are networking, multiple contacts, and persistence.

69 Urgent care centers

Dentists who add sports dentistry to their practices, says Ray R. Padilla, DDS, West Covina, CA, should make themselves available for emergency trauma care. "They can do this," he suggests, "by contacting local pediatricians, urgent care centers, hospital emergency rooms, and schools to let them know they're available for trauma therapy."

"Dentists can also make themselves visible and available," adds Dr. Padilla, "to coaches, sports physicians, trainers, sports therapists, PTA and booster groups, health clubs, youth sports leagues, and women's athletics. Dentists can offer to speak at organization meetings, attend their games or events, and develop mutual trust and credibility through community involvement."[8]

Another source of potential referrals is hotel concierges.

FROM THE SUCCESS FILES

In the early days of his practice, Andrew C. Doerfler, DDS, Spring, TX, formed an alliance with nearby dentists for the purpose of contacting school nurses and offering their services to indigent children with dental emergencies at school. This alliance resulted in several such patients.

This kindness, however, also led several school nurses to become patients of Dr. Doerfler as well as referral sources for both students and teachers.

70 Diabetologists, endocrinologists, and internists

"The dentist plays a pivotal role in managing the diabetic patient," says Anthony T. Vernillo, DDS, PhD, in *Global Health Nexus*, a publication of New York University College of Dentistry. "As part of the healthcare team, the dentist's goal is controlling the patient's diabetes through prevention."[9]

"Understanding the role of nutrition in the care of diabetics is important, and the dental team needs to interact more frequently with diabetologists, endocrinologists, and internists who treat diabetics, so that the quality of care provided to the diabetic patient continues to improve," says D. Walter Cohen, DDS, Dean Emeritus, University of Pennsylvania School of Dental Medicine. "The results of information sharing among dentists and physicians will benefit both patients and the dental profession, which will achieve yet another advance in the area of prevention."[10]

REALITY CHECK

"The risk of developing Type 2 diabetes, osteoporosis, and heart disease increases with age," writes Craig W. Valentine, DMD, FAGD, Lakeland, FL, national spokesperson for the AGD. "Researchers believe that these diseases often manifest themselves in the mouth, making dentists a key player in diagnosis."[11]

71 Podiatrists

Podiatrists, who are often the primary point of care for people with diabetes, are aware of the need for a comprehensive, multidisciplinary approach to care—including periodic visits to a dentist. Consider the following excerpt from the article "Taking Ownership of Your Patients with Diabetes" by Ross E. Taubmann, DPM, from *Podiatry Management* magazine.

"Each person with diabetes should know that an often-overlooked component of diabetes complications is oral health. Of particular concern are the effects of diabetes on the gingival and periodontal tissues. Additionally, there can be symptoms of diabetic neuropathy, fungal infections, and tooth decay caused by diabetes. It is important for podiatrists to remind patients to conduct a monthly self-examination of their teeth and oral cavity. In addition, inquire if your patients are seeing their dental professionals regularly, at least once every six months. If a patient is not receiving appropriate oral health-care, a podiatrist should encourage and refer them to oral healthcare providers."[12]

ACTION STEPS

The groundwork has been done. Touch base with podiatrists in your community. Establish a dialogue based on your overlapping interest in monitoring, preventing, and treating diabetes. It will lead to improved patient care and reciprocal referrals.

72 Pharmacists

There are numerous topics of mutual interest to dentists and pharmacists. These include diabetes as well as prescription and over-the-counter drugs and other oral health products.

Of importance also is the fact that pharmacists are frequently asked by their patrons for advice about oral hygiene products, over-the-counter medications for minor dental problems, and more than you might guess, for the name of a good dentist.

FROM THE SUCCESS FILES

When periodontist Mitchell T. Cantor, DMD, MSD, first opened his practice in Southampton, Long Island, NY, he mailed individual letters to local pharmacists and enclosed a list of oral hygiene devices recommended by his office. The hope was that these items or their equivalent would be kept in stock and available to his patients. The letter ended with "We will be glad to answer any questions you have."

Such a letter is an effective, low-key way to start the process of networking.

73 Nursing homes, assisted living facilities, and senior centers

"There continues to be a shortage of dentists providing care to those elderly who are homebound or in nursing homes," says Barry W. Ceridan, DDS, Louisville, KY, past president of the American Society of Geriatric Dentistry.[13]

"Have you ever viewed your ability to answer an adult son or daughter's request to perform a dental consult on Mom or Dad in a nursing home as a form of marketing?" asks Linda C. Niessen, DMD, MPH, clinical professor in the department of public health sciences at Baylor College of Dentistry-Texas A&M University System, Dallas, TX. "It's true that answering a nursing home consult will take additional time in your already busy life. Keep in mind, however, that you and your dental team will be viewed as caring, committed professionals when you answer that request. And once in the nursing home, you have the opportunity to educate the healthcare staff, physicians, nurses, nurses' aides, occupational therapists, etc., on the importance of oral health throughout life."[14]

ACTION STEP

"Partner with a local nursing home, assisted living facility, or senior center," says Lori Trost, DMD, editor of *Woman Dentist Journal*. "These delightful people appreciate your energy, time and information. Explain the benefits of rinses, cleansers, nutrition, and continued periodontal maintenance. Everyone benefits—you, you team, your practice, and your community."[15]

RESOURCES

Two helpful publications are available from the American Dental Association: Providing Dental Care in Long-Term Care Facilities: A Resource Manual (Catalog number J010) and Non-Traditional Practice Settings: Developing New Ways to Practice Dentistry (Catalog number J017); www.adacatalog.org or (800)-947-4746.

74 Establish a referral network

Write selected physicians in your community. Explain that you're in the process of establishing a network of primary care physicians and specialists to whom you can refer patients who are new in the area or without a physician. And request information about *their* practices.

Keep such a letter *low-key*. Do not include a brochure about your practice, article reprints, or business cards.

LEARNED LESSON

Working with only your own interests in mind will not work. Aggressive networking turns people off because it fails to establish trust.

REALITY CHECK

The response to such a letter will depend on a number of factors including: how swamped the physician's practice is with patients, the perceived sincerity of your letter (i.e., whether or not it appears self-serving), and perhaps even the stationery on which it is written. In some cases, such letters have opened doors, prompted physicians to pick up the phone, request further information and, down the line, resulted in reciprocal referrals.

FROM THE SUCCESS FILES

"Our directory of physicians and allied health care professionals," says Albert Ousbourne, DDS, Towson, MD, "has consistently proven to produce reciprocal referrals."

75 The secret of a successful specialist–general practitioner relationship

"To be successful, you must create a climate of understanding between you and the GP," advises The American Academy of Periodontology in its publication *Ideas to Help Your Practice Grow*. "This means really *understanding* what appeals to him or her so you can work out a referral plan that benefits you both. For example, strive to understand and ask each GP outright the following questions:"

"What is your treatment philosophy?"

"What type of communication do you prefer? How frequently would you like to hear from me?"

"How would you want me to handle a non-compliant patient or one who doesn't wish to return to you for treatment?"

"How do you see my treatment plan fitting into your overall restorative vision?"

"What are your overall goals for patient health?"
"Do you perceive me as working 'with' or 'against' you?"[16]

HARD-LEARNED LESSON
"Make sure you and the specialist agree on guidelines for appropriate and timely referrals," says A. Steven Gutter, DDS, Aventura, FL. "The last thing either dentist wants is a patient asking, 'Why wasn't I referred earlier?' Review clinical criteria together and be sure you're both comfortable with each other's best practice philosophies."[17]

76 Why general practitioners refer to specialists

Arthur Goldenburg, DDS, an endodontist in White Plains, NY, conducted a survey in the Ninth District Dental Society (New York) and the Danbury, Connecticut Dental Society. Of the 102 surveys returned, 72 were from general dentists. Among the results:

- 90% felt that referrals were based on competence.
- 53% refer because of friendships.
- 75% refer because of reputation.
- 66% heard the specialist speak and therefore refer (see Secret #41).

"Referrals," concluded Dr. Goldenberg, "are not made on gifts the specialist buys for the referring dentist, socializing with spouses, or a year-end party. The overall impression is that contact between practitioners and specialists must be sincere, not aggressive, overbearing, or overly frequent."[18]

REALITY CHECK
"A computer-generated form letter from a specialist thanking me for a referral," a GP told me, "is a real turnoff."

77 Win-win strategies

The most effective networking strategies are those that are *mutually beneficial,* such as inviting GPs to a seminar hosted by your office on clinical or practice management topics.

Presenting a program on a topic such as "Diagnosis and Treatment Planning for the Implant Patient" (by yourself or an outside speaker) greatly benefits those attending. It enhances their knowledge and clinical skills and, at the same time, increases their referral potential. Presenting it yourself has the added advantage of showcasing your clinical expertise and philosophy of practice to a wide audience.

"Many specialists are learning that the more a general dentist knows about a particular specialty," says William H. Howard, DMD, MAGD, the more a general dentist is likely to refer patients."[19]

Practice management topics presented by nationally known speakers not only draw large numbers of GPs, but also their staff members. This gives your staff members a unique opportunity to network with their counterparts in the audience—an added plus for their working relationships.

Another consideration: educational programs for GPs that are held at upscale hotels and country clubs with a nice luncheon or wine and cheese get-together (after the program) are enjoyable networking opportunities for everyone. They're also a "classy" way to express appreciation to GPs for their continued support and referrals.

TESTED TIP

Worded properly, the letter inviting referring dentists to a specialist-sponsored seminar can be part of the relationship-building process. For example, the following are the opening paragraphs of two such letters for programs at which I was the invited speaker. The first is from an orthodontist, the second from an orthodontist and a periodontist who co-sponsored the program.

- "I want to take this opportunity to thank you sincerely for the support that you have given me over the years in the form of referrals. The main purpose of this letter is just to let you know that I don't take this support for granted, but rather I appreciate it fully for what it represents. And I want you to know that I will do everything I can to deserve this in the future."

- "This year Ellen and I have decided to express our gratitude to the dentists like yourself who have supported us so well over the last few years. Instead of Christmas parties or baskets of fruit, we are sponsoring a seminar by a noted speaker who will be addressing a subject that is important to all of us."

These were only the opening paragraphs of the two letters. The body of each letter then went on to describe the details of the program and registration.

78 Newsletters to referring doctors

Donald Hayden, MD, a dermatologist in Oceanside, CA, developed a newsletter for referral sources entitled *What's New in Dermatology*. The first issue had the following cover letter:

Dear Colleague,

This newsletter is being sent to you with the hope it will provide helpful information for you on the newest developments in dermatology. It's also a "thank you" for the confidence you have shown by referring patients to us.
    If you have any questions regarding dermatology, please don't hesitate to call. I am most happy to help you in any way I can in the management and care of your patients.

Sincerely,

Many dental specialists have similarly used newsletters to network with their referring dentists. Some include in such newsletters a "guest columnist" from their network along with his or her resume and a photograph. This makes the newsletter more interesting and informative. It's also a great way to cement a referral relationship.

FROM THE SUCCESS FILES
"When I find media articles that talk about the effect of periodontal health on total health," says periodontist Douglas M. Neuman, DMD,

gton, KY, "I have these articles laminated and then give them to general dentists to use with their patients."

---

79 Lunch and learn

"Create a 30-minute slide presentation on the topics of aesthetic crown lengthening and gingival recession," suggests periodontist Roberta L. Shaklee, DDS, Denver, CO. "Then offer to conduct a 30-minute slide show during the lunch hour—when general dentistry offices typically hold staff meetings—and provide boxed lunches for the referring dentist and staff."

"This approach," says Dr. Shaklee, "will provide continuing education for referring dentists and their staffs and enable them to become better acquainted with you. Educating the dental hygienist is important because the patient often spends more time with the hygienist than the doctor. The hygienist can discuss the benefits of aesthetic periodontal treatment with the patient."[20]

FROM THE SUCCESS FILES

"More orthodontists are seeking referrals from the staffs of referring doctors," write practice management consultant Martin L. "Bud" Schulman and John K. McGill. "As general dentists have become busier with a wider array of services to their ever growing patient base, they are less inclined to 'look for' patients that may need orthodontic treatment. Many successful orthodontists have been very effective in targeting hygienists through continuing education programs and luncheons with their staff members to have them suggest orthodontic treatment to the doctor or directly to the patient."[21]

---

80 Network with "the influentials"

Word-of-mouth recommendations about your practice are far more convincing, credible, and persuasive than any form of *self-promotion* or *paid advertising* designed to obtain new patients. That's a given.

Not all word-of-mouth recommendations, however, are equivalent. Some referral sources are *more* convincing, credible, and persuasive than others. *The Influentials* are one such group.

Who are they?

Ed Keller and Jon Berry, CEO and vice president, respectively, of global marketing research and consulting firm Roper-ASW, are authors of *The Influentials*. They report that Influential Americans represent roughly 10% of the adult population. That figure translates into 5000 people in every city with 50,000 people 18 or older and, on a national level, 21 million people.

They live up to their name as people who actively influence others. They're highly regarded, trusted, and regularly asked for advice on all kinds of questions, both personal and professional. Their influence is most important for services that depend on word-of-mouth recommendation, like healthcare.

Keller and Berry define an Influential American as someone who has done three or more of the following in the past year: attended a public meeting, written a legislator, been an officer or committee member of a local organization, attended a political speech or rally, made a speech, written a letter to the editor or called a live radio or TV show to express an opinion, worked for a political party, worked for an activist group, written an article, or held or run for political office.

Influential Americans are predominantly in their 30s and 40s and married with children. They are wealthier, better educated, hold higher-level jobs, and are more time-pressured than most Americans. They put a priority on health and fitness. Of 14 exercise activities ranging from calisthenics to swimming, 86% of Influentials do at least one of them on a regular basis.

This combination of education, activity, and high income gives these influential people "an insatiable thirst for knowledge and information," says Tom Miller, senior vice president at the Roper Organization. According to their studies, the more information and less "hard sell" you give these influential people, the better your chances of persuading them.

TRENDSETTERS

Pioneer consumers. Trendsetters. Bellwether consumers. Leading-edge buyers. Experimenters. Early adopters. All of these terms have been used to describe Influential Americans, because this group leads the pack in accepting new products and activities.

uentials popularized digital cameras, for example, long before their neighbors knew what they were. "By early 2001," Keller and Berry say, "one in six Influentials owned a digital camera (double the rate of the public as a whole) and a comparable proportion were planning to buy one in the next year or two (more than double the public as a whole). Three in ten had viewed personal photos over a computer in the past month, about triple the rate of the total public. The net effect pointed to an increasingly digital future for photography. Good news for companies selling digital cameras and software to help people archive, edit, transmit, and tinker with their digital photo collections."[22]

REALITY CHECK

State-of-the-art equipment, cutting-edge technology, and the newest innovations in restorative and cosmetic dentistry would by definition resonate if not strongly appeal to such patients.

The critical point is that Influential Americans are typically trendsetters, and their acceptance or rejection of a product or service can mean the difference between success and failure.

If you're involved with networking, it's a group you definitely want to reach.

WHERE TO FIND THEM

Keller and Berry write that Influential Americans are social butterflies. They are avid communicators on a personal level and enthusiastic patrons of social activities, whether they're entertaining friends at home, attending church get-togethers, going out to a nightclub, or writing, telephoning, or e-mailing a family member. They're nearly four times as likely as average Americans to attend meetings of a club or civic organization, and such activities greatly extend their sphere of influence.

Perhaps most significant, Influentials carry more weight in the marketplace than their numbers and buying power would suggest. The reason is that people trust them and ask them for advice. Keller and Berry report that these people are two, three, or four times more likely than the average person to be asked for advice on a particular product or service, and are much more likely to give advice concerning such topics as health, government, politics, children, restaurants, computers, insurance, investments, cars, sports, art, and music.

Making a good impression on just one Influential American, they say, can create *six* brand loyal customers. It's reasonable to assume their professional referrals have an equal amount of clout.

INFLUENTIALS TAKE ACTION

Keller and Berry indicate that Influentials hold high standards for quality and performance, and will take action if they're dissatisfied. They tend to complain more readily, and they'll stop buying a product or leave a service provider if they're disappointed. They'll also broadcast a negative experience to their wide network of friends and colleagues. "Influentials, a crowd easily given to action," they say, "are an unfortunate group to alienate with poor quality or poor service."[22]

ACTION STEP

If you're interested in increasing the numbers and clout of your referral sources, consider networking with Influential Americans in the kinds of activities in which they are actively engaged, and be sure to address their needs and priorities in your practice.

---

81 Hard-learned lessons about networking

It's important to realize that networking is not an "entitlement program" in which you are eligible for referrals because you want or need them. It's not giving away business cards and asking for referrals.

A thirty-something dentist spoke for many GPs I've interviewed when he said, "I resent the invitations to lunch so frequently extended by specialists. The unspoken purpose is obvious: referrals. To put it bluntly," he added, "my referrals aren't for sale."

Networking is not a quick fix for an ailing practice or shortage of patients. Relationships require nurturing and a long-term outlook, more like farming than manufacturing.

Some dentists make these initial networking contacts, perhaps exchange information and, if it doesn't generate immediate referrals, they give up on the idea. "Been there. Done that," they say. What they recognize is that networking is an ongoing process, not a one-time event.

In the words of urologist Neil Baum, MD, New Orleans, LA, the cultivation of physician referrals takes "patience, persistence, and prompt reporting."

Corollary: "The biggest mistake for a specialist to make," says the *Blair/McGill Advisory*, "is to let your patient beat your referral back to the referring doctor. In that situation, your referrer has no input for the next patient visit, and worse yet, may be surprised or embarrassed, and thus directly reminded of your inattentiveness. That's a sure-fire way to lose referrals."[23]

Notes

1. Zwerling F, Zwerling MH. On Finding Success in Practice. *Medical Economics,* February 2001, 1997, 97.
2. Poss SD. How to Profit from Endodontics. *Dental Economics,* February 1999.
3. Kossak ME. The Physician Referral. *The Personal Report,* April 1992, 21.
4. Dorfman WM. The Ultimate Dental Product—Your Practice. *Dental Products Report,* June 1997, 58-61.
5. Hedge T. Dentistry and the Extreme Makeover. *Dental Economics,* September 2003, 54-56.
6. Mouth Gives "Warning Signs" of Larger Health Problems. *Dentistry Today,* July 2003, 26.
7. Simon J. No Caries . . . No Perio . . . Could the Fellow Below Use a Dentist? *Dental Economics,* May 2003, 52-55.
8. Padilla RR. Sports in Daily Practice. *Academy of Sports Dentistry,* August, 1997, 13, 2, 4.
9. Vernillo AT. Practice for Life: The Dentist's Role in Managing the Diabetic Patient, *Global Health Nexus,* Summer 2003, 5, 2, 16-17.
10. Cohen DW. Diabetes and Oral Health: A Call to Action. *Global Health Nexus,* College of Dentistry, New York University, Summer 2003, 5, 2, 7-11.
11. Valentine CW. Talking to Baby Boomers. *Dental Equipment & Materials,* January/February 2004, 38-39.
12. Taubman RE. Taking Ownership of Your Patients With Diabetes. *Podiatry Management,* November 2002, 77-78.
13. McKee L. Opportunities to help others, build practice found in nursing homes. *ADA News,* March 2, 1998, 19, 24.
14. Niessen LC. Customers for Life: Marketing Oral Health Care to Older Adults. *Dental Economics,* August 2000, 142-147.
15. Trost L. Editor's Note: Matters of the Heart. *Woman Dentist Journal,* February 2004, 6.
16. Ideas to Help Your Practice Grow. *The American Academy of Periodontology,* 1995, 8.
17. Gutter AS. Take Time to Nurture Successful Referral Relationships. *Dental Practice Advisor,* April 2000, 1, 3.

18. Smith C. Two's Company, But Three's Not a Crowd. *AGD Impact,* January 1999, 10-15.
19. Howard WH. Editorial. *AGD Impact,* April 1996.
20. Shaklee RL. Increasing Your Referral Base by Marketing Esthetic Periodontal Procedures. *AAP News,* September/October 2000.
21. Schulman ML, McGill JK. *How Does Your Orthodontic Practice Stack Up? Blair/McGill Advisory.* February 2002, 2-3.
22. Keller E, Berry J. *The Influential Americans.* New York: The Free Press, 2003.
23. Mistakes in Reporting Back to Referring Doctors. *Blair/McGill Advisory,* March 1998, 4.

7

Patient Expectations, Satisfaction, and Loyalty

In a *Fast Company* article, Lucy McCauley asks, "You already know that the customer is always right, right? But these days—given the speed and interactivity of the Internet, the explosion of customer choice, the emergence of new competitive pressures, and the constant expansion of customers' expectations for service—just giving customers what they want isn't enough. You also have to anticipate needs, solve problems before they start, provide service that wows, and offer responses to mistakes that more than make up for the original error."[1]

The article was aimed at the business community. But it's also dead-on for dentistry.

82 Patient loyalty

Let's start with some approximations of patient loyalty based on practice surveys I've done throughout the country.

Fiercely loyal dental patients who are not likely to switch to another office make up 10%-30% of patients surveyed.

Another 25%-50% are more or less inclined to stay with the same dentist or specialist. Unlike the first grouping, they can be, and often are, "lured" away by other offices.

Finally, 10%-25% really don't care where they go or whom they see. They tend to view dentistry or orthodontics or the other specialties as *commodities*, and select them strictly on price or convenience or because a provider is listed in a directory from a managed care plan.

What are the secrets of earning the goodwill of patients who are in that fiercely loyal group?

83 The expectations gap

Our studies indicate that in the typical practice, 75% of referrals are made by only 15%-20% of patients. Why so few? The answer lies in what I call the "Expectations Gap" or the disparity between a patient's *expectations* about a visit to a dentist and his or her *perception* of the experience itself.

It's an oversimplification to be sure, but for the sake of discussion let's divide the patients in a typical practice into three groups, starting with the least happy.

1. The first group is those patients who are *disappointed* by the experience of a visit to a dental office because their expectations for quality of care, office environment, punctuality, a friendly staff, and the like were *not met*. These are *dissatisfied* patients who, depending on the severity of their complaints, may take several courses of action.
   - Mildly dissatisfied patients usually say nothing at the time. Most tolerate minor shortcomings—but less so if they occur on a repeated basis.
   - Patients with greater dissatisfaction speak up. In many cases, they repeat the story of what went wrong to their friends, acquaintances, and perhaps their co-workers. Such negative word-of-mouth can seriously damage your reputation and referrals. If such patients were referred by a dental colleague, physician, or other professional, the bad reports can possibly *end* that referral relationship.
   - Truly *angry* patients leave the practice, possibly notify their managed care plan administrator and, in the worst-case scenario, sue for malpractice.

Many of these cases sprout from a communication breakdown between dentists and patients, says John Vaselaney, DDS, national director of the dental risk management program for CNA HealthPro in Chicago. "It's not bad dentistry that's causing these lawsuits," he adds, "it's bad communication."[2]

2. The second group is those patients whose expectations were *essentially met*. "The doctor was OK." "The hygienist was OK." "The office was OK." These are *satisfied* patients. Many patients use the word "satisfaction" (or "OK"), not so much to express positive feelings but rather to communicate the absence of negative feelings. It often turns out to be a "neutral" feeling that means they may or may not talk about their experience. They may or may not refer anyone. They may or may not even *stay* in the practice.

3. The third group of patients is those whose expectations for quality of care, office environment, and so on are *more than met*. They're *exceeded*! When asked about their experience, these patients talk in glowing terms about the "the most thorough exam I've ever had," "the high-tech office," "the thoughtfulness of the staff," and on and on. Their experience was more than "OK." They're more than satisfied. More than just "happy." These are *enthusiastic* patients, the ones who make *referrals*, who convince other family members to come to you, who *thank* the friend or physician or whoever referred them, *and* who pay their bills cheerfully and promptly. Even more important, these patients are intensely *loyal*. They'll stick with you, whether or not you're a provider on their managed care plan, or have higher fees, or keep them waiting.

In the *typical* practice, these enthusiastic patients represent the 15-20% of patients who account for 75% of referrals.

High-performance dental practices, on the other hand, have a higher-than-average number of enthusiastic, loyal patients and, in turn, a higher-than-average number of referrals. The reason is simple: patients' expectations are greatly exceeded—not just once in a while, but on every visit.

REALITY CHECK

The following are findings of Technical Assistance Research Programs, Inc. (TARP), a 30-year-old consumer satisfaction and consulting firm headquartered in Arlington, VA.

- "About two-thirds of dental patients dissatisfied with the quality of care at their office are not likely to complain to dental staff," says Daniel McCann, senior editor at *Dental Practice Report*. "Reasons given include: 'It's not worth the bother,' 'It won't have any effect,' and 'Fear that I might be treated poorly during my next visit.'"
- "Between 50 and 90 percent of these people will go elsewhere for future care."
- "Dissatisfied patients typically relate their complaint to between four and eight people. And compared to positive reports about a practitioner, negative comments are twice as likely to influence a prospective patient looking for a dentist."[3]

84 Process versus outcome

Patients typically use two criteria to evaluate their overall experience: *process* and *outcome*. Both must match the patient's expectations to be judged satisfactory. Both must exceed expectations to be viewed as outstanding. If either falls short of the patient's expectations, it will result in a negative experience. Consider the following example:

If the outcome (the crown or dental prophylaxis, for example) is wonderful but the patient's experience (the process) was painful or upsetting in any way, the overall evaluation will be negative.

In the same way, if you and your staff provide five-star service but fall short (in the patient's mind) on the quality of care, the evaluation will again be negative.

What this means is that the caring is as important as the care itself in exceeding patients' expectations and winning their loyalty. Both are important.

FROM THE SUCCESS FILES

"A number of years ago," recalls Debra Gray King, DDS, FAACD, president of the Atlanta (Georgia) Center for Cosmetic Dentistry, "our practice envisioned a world in which a visit to the dentist is relaxing, pampering . . . a treat. Would people actually look forward to getting their regular checkups? Would they go ahead and get that Hollywood smile they always wanted? We discovered the answer is a resounding 'yes!'"

"As we realized how quickly our patients embraced the initial pampering changes in our practice," Dr. King adds, "we focused on making the dental visit even more stress-free, restful, and, yes, even enjoyable. We wanted the treatment to be so pleasant, so antithetical to what the average person expects from a dental visit, that it actually creates an army of ambassadors and raving fans. We wanted patients not only to love their new smile, but actually enjoy the process of getting it."[4]

REALITY CHECK

"Who defines quality?" asks Kenneth C. Jones, writing in the *Journal of Health Care Finance.* "Consumers are not able to measure quality the same way that healthcare providers measure it, as they do not usually have the technical capability to evaluate what was provided. Patients define quality through factors such as the quality of the relationship with the caregiver, not the quality of the clinical care. Providers need to educate caregivers on the importance of explaining what the patient is about to experience and to answer questions fully. The caregiver needs to build trust, respect, and encourage communication. Caregivers must be reliable, prompt, and helpful."

"The perception of quality and consumer satisfaction," Mr. Jones says, "is created in how care is provided."[5]

---

85 The civility factor

Yankelovich Partners Inc., one of the premier market research firms in the United States, specializes in studying consumer behavior and attitudes, often the best predictor of future marketplace behavior. Their signature product *Monitor®* is an ongoing survey of 2500 consumers. These consumers, 16 years and older from all parts of the country, are interviewed in their homes for 2 hours. They're asked hundreds of questions about their values, beliefs, and behaviors on a wide variety of topics, for example, "What is most important to you regarding customer service—that is, the way you are treated by business or its employees when purchasing products or services?"[6]

The following are the results in descending order:

Courtesy	25%
Knowledgeable	21%
Friendliness	13%
Listens to you	13%
Efficiency	10%
Thoroughness	8%
Promptness	5%
Availability	5%

What's interesting about these findings is that *efficiency,* often the focus of dentists' efforts to improve the profitability of their practices, is significantly less important to consumers than courtesy, friendliness, and simply being listened to.

Britt Beemer, author of *Predatory Marketing*, isn't surprised by these statistics. "Efficiency is not a replacement for customer service," he says. "It's only a small part of building relationships with customers. This blind focus on efficiency perfectly describes the breach between what customers want and what companies think they want."[7]

"The overriding message of these findings," Barbara Kaplan, a partner at Yankelovich Partners, Inc., told me, "is that people want to be treated with *civility*. If they're not, they can and will go elsewhere."

The "civility factor," as I now call it, should be an important consideration when deciding whom to hire and what the priorities of your practice will be.

FROM THE SUCCESS FILES

In a 2003 nationwide study of hospitals published by AARP *Modern Maturity,* North Shore University Hospital, Manhasset, NY, was selected as the number one hospital in America.[8]

After patients' visits to the hospital's emergency department, a survey is sent to their homes. It asks for feedback about their visits; interactions with admitting personnel, doctors, and nurses; and how (if they were accompanied) their family or friends were treated. Only three to five questions are asked about each, requesting patients to "rank their experience" on a scale of one to five (very poor to very good).

What's significant is that every cluster of questions about interactions included a question about *courtesy* as the first question (e.g., the courtesy of the nurses, the doctor, the person who took your blood, the radiology staff, the person who took your personal/insurance information, and the courtesy with which family or friends were treated).

HARD-LEARNED LESSON

"One of the lessons to be learned about service," say consultants Karl Albrecht and Lawrence J. Bradford, PhD, "is that the longer a business has been in existence, the more likely it is that it has lost sight of what is important to customers."[9]

86 Learn new patients' expectations

REALITY CHECK

"For almost every business," says George Columbo, author of *Killer Customer Care: How to Provide Five star Service That Will Double and Triple Your Profits,* "a whole set of unconscious or 'hidden' expectations affect the quality of its customers' experiences. If you focus only on the most explicit expectations, then your customers' experiences will almost certainly be much less satisfying than possible. Sure you must address your customers' primary expectations," he adds, "but you should also be tenaciously trying to understand all of your customers' expectations—especially the hidden ones—and then exploring ways to address them all."[10]

ACTION STEPS

The key to uncovering a patient's real expectations is asking open-ended questions, says Irwin Becker, DDS, Education Chairman of the Pankey Institute. You need to hear much more than "Yes," "No," or "Well, it hurts when I bite down" before you can design, let alone persuade the patient to accept a comprehensive treatment plan. So frame questions and comments to solicit information about the following issues:

- How highly does the patient value oral health?
- What past experiences have influenced patient attitudes about oral health and dentistry?
- What does the patient believe is his or her biggest dental problem?

- How important to the patient is resolving that problem?
- What has prevented this patient from dealing with the problem before now?
- What does the patient expect you to do for him or her?
- What does the patient really want you to do for him or her?
- How willing is the patient to make a long-term commitment to better oral health?

Your objective, notes Dr. Becker, is to get the patient talking. Don't commandeer the interview with clinical explanations. Remember, "People make more decisions when they hear themselves talk than when listening to you." Encourage the patient to carry 80% of the discussion. Prompt gently only when necessary to stay on track. Your role is helping patients clarify for themselves real and perceived needs.[11]

REALITY CHECK

"The most common mistake made by periodontists/surgeons," says periodontist Perry Klokkevold, DDS, and restorative colleague, George Perri, DDS, "is proceeding with implant therapy without a good understanding of the patient's desires, restorative treatment goals, and restorative limitations of the case. Do not hesitate to call the patient and/or referring doctors to clarify anything that is unclear. The communication you offer will be well received, greatly appreciated, and go a long way in preventing much anxiety and avoiding unnecessary headaches."[12]

---

87 Manage patients' expectations

Patients often have unrealistic expectations. Take managed care, for example. Some patients have the mistaken belief that everything about treatment will be the same as before, except cheaper, possibly even free. All they'll ever have to pay is a nominal co-payment for office visits.

Healthcare practitioners address this problem by communicating plan rules with their patients from the start of the relationship. They manage their patients' expectations, telling them what to expect, what they can and cannot do in seeking treatment, and generally how the new system works. In most cases, it lowers expectations to more realistic levels.

FROM THE SUCCESS FILES

Catherine Martin, business administrator at the office of Roberta Cann, DMD, Atlanta, GA, says she has to educate patients about their insurance coverage. "We're a very high-end practice that charges a high fee for crown and bridge," she says, adding that many patients assume their insurance company will pay 50% of the procedure no matter what. "I have to explain that our fees are not the usual and customary, so even if the insurance company pays between $400 and $500, the patient may be responsible for $800 out pocket."[13]

"In our office," says Steve Lynch, DMD, Oxford, AL, "we don't wait until patients are in the chair before we begin to manage expectations. We start as soon as they come through the door by using digital radiography to help sell them on our way of dentistry. Our digital X-ray system is one of the most important marketing tools in our office. A team member in my office explains to each new patient that we have digital radiography and it's one way we help improve patient outcomes for dental treatment. That's the beginning of managing expectations—*creating* them in the first place. We want our patients to expect the safest and best treatment."[14]

88 Hard-learned lessons about unrealistic expectations

"Experienced implant dentists," says Paul Homoly, DDS, Holt, MI, "have learned to under-promise and over-deliver. This attitude goes beyond informed-consent procedures. There's no amount of consent that can douse the flames of discontent of patients who believe they were misled." Quoting implant practitioner, Dr. Kim Gowey, he adds, "Patients with unrealistic, uncompromising expectations are best left untreated."[15]

"We try to determine if a patient's expectations are beyond what we feel we can do," says Larry Rosenthal, DDS, New York, NY, who has built an international reputation for his expertise in aesthetic dentistry.

"For patients with unrealistic expectations, we try to make them understand that this may not be the office for them."[16]

"The most important thing a dentist can do is determine a patient's expectations prior to the start of treatment," says Wynn Okuda, DMD, Honolulu, HI, past president of the American Academy of Dentistry. "I spend a lot of time consulting with the patient, and find it critical to my success. Patients need to know the options (for tooth whitening). They also need to know if bleaching will meet their expectations. Patients have expectations about the end result. If those expectations are met, they are going to say a lot of positive things about cosmetic dentistry. However, patients have to understand there are limitations of bleaching. In my experience, teeth heavily stained by tetracycline will revert and relapse a significant number of times after bleaching. Ultimately, these people have to go to other cosmetic dental procedures such as composite or porcelain veneers. There are times I recommend going straight to veneers knowing whitening will not meet their expectations."[17]

89 Your top 50

Do you know the identity of the 50 best patients in your practice? Those who have been in the practice the longest? Who bring their entire families to you? Make the most referrals? Spend the most on your services? Does your staff know them?

Imagine the following scenario: one of the top 50 calls your practice, identifies herself, requests an appointment, and is asked by the receptionist, "Are you a patient here?"

ACTION STEPS

Hold a staff meeting to decide the top 50 patients in your practice, using whatever criteria you think are relevant. If you have a really large practice, go for the top 100. If smaller, target the top 20. These are your practice's movers and shakers.

Keep a list at the front desk. Put an easy-to-spot code on their record or computer file. And give these patients extra special treatment at every opportunity. Juggle your schedule if necessary, to arrange ntments at their convenience, or come in early or stay late to accommodate them. Go to whatever lengths necessary to give them the best possible service. See them on time. Provide personalized attention. And if your receptionist doesn't recognize the name of a caller, instead of asking, "Are you a patient here?" suggest she ask, "When did you last see the doctor?"

REALITY CHECK

In the best of all worlds, every patient deserves V.I.P. treatment. However, the peaks and valleys of most practices make that difficult. So start with the top 50.

---

90 Strive for patient loyalty

"One of the biggest mistakes we've made in the past," says Tim Banker, DVM, Greensboro, NC, "is to take loyal clients for granted, while spinning our wheels trying to get new clients. We now let loyal clients know how much we appreciate them."

There are many benefits (beyond the obvious) of having loyal patients.

Loyal patients by definition have more trust in the recommendations made by dentists, hygienists, and staff members. They tend to come in more often and spend more per visit.

Loyal patients tend to be more tolerant of minor problems, delays, and the like.

Loyal patients are the most vocal in telling others about the quality of care and service they received. "In fact," says Frederick F. Reichheld, author of *Loyalty Rules!* "such a recommendation is one of the best indicators of loyalty because of the customer's sacrifice, if you will, in making the recommendation. When customers act as references, they do more than indicate they've received good economic value from a company; they put their own reputations on the line. And they will risk their own reputations only if they feel intense loyalty."[18]

Revenue grows as a result of repeat visits, purchases, and referrals.

Costs decline as a result of the efficiencies of seeing "experienced" patients who require less paperwork and explanations.

Costs also decline as the needs for advertising and practice promotion decrease. (It costs 5 times more to acquire a new patient than it does to retain an existing one.)

Employee retention increases because of job pride and satisfaction, which in turn create a loop that reinforces patient loyalty and further reduces costs as hiring and training costs decrease and productivity rises.

As costs go down and revenues go up, *profitability* increases.

REALITY CHECK

"In short, increased customer loyalty is the single most important driver of long-term profitability," say Scott Robinette, president of the Hallmark Loyalty Group, a division of Hallmark Cards Inc., and Claire Brand, General Manager of Hallmark Keepsakes.[19]

FROM THE SUCCESS FILES

Frank A. Zampieri, DDS, Fort Lee, NJ, sends out silver Tiffany pens to patients who have been in his practice for 25 years. He estimates that he has sent out more than 100 pens, which is a testament to his relationship with his patients.[20]

91 Retention versus loyalty

Patient retention is not the same thing as patient loyalty. If you're the only dentist in town, you'll retain your patients. Suppose, however, other practices open in your area. Will your patients remain loyal?

Loyalty implies a *choice*. It's a very important distinction.

"Core service doesn't generate loyalty," says Stephanie A. Busty, a training specialist at New York City's Beth Israel Hospital. "It's getting the service up to extraordinary levels. We want to exceed expectations. We want to knock their socks off."[21]

REALITY CHECK

Bob Kornfeld, DPM, Lake Success, NY, recounts a story that unfortunately is all too familiar.

"I moved only 6 miles from an office I ran for over 18 years. After moving, we experienced a 65 percent loss of all of the local patients.

It took 3 years to build the volume back to what it had previously been. In that time, we have had some of those former patients return here (10 minutes from the other office) but overall, lost 55 percent of the locals. To be perfectly honest, I was shocked when it happened. I convinced myself I was worth the 10 minute car ride. But patients have a different agenda and to them, convenience is obviously the priority."[22]

92 Word-of-mouth wins!

"The best marketing," says Larry Rosenthal, DDS, Director of the New York Group for Aesthetic Dentistry in New York City, "is word-of-mouth."[23]

"The American public has long known the value of word-of-mouth recommendations," say Ed Keller and Jon Berry, chief executive and vice president of Roper-ASW. "According to Roper research, Americans today are far more likely to turn to friends, family, and other personal experts than to use traditional media for ideas and information on a range of topics. We know," Keller and Berry say, "because on a regular basis for 25 years, we've been asking people which of a variety of sources—TV programs, TV commercials, newspaper stories, newspaper ads, magazine stories, magazine ads, online or Internet sources, friends, family, or other people—give them the best ideas and information on different decisions. For information about healthcare, hotels to stay in, merits of cars, computer equipment, and a host of other issues, Americans generally are *twice as likely* to cite word of mouth as the best source of ideas and information in these and other areas as they are to cite advertising."[24]

They're not alone in reaching this conclusion.

"According to a McKinsey & Co. study, 67 percent of U.S. consumer goods sales are based on word-of-mouth. Heavy exposure to the best and most expensive advertising is not enough to get people to part with their money, whereas a mere mention of a product by friends, family, even strangers will often do the trick."[25]

"Affluent individuals," says Thomas J. Stanley, author of *Networking with the Affluent,* "report that word-of-mouth endorsements are the most influential in their decisions to patronize a variety of product and service providers."

FROM THE SUCCESS FILES
"You will be surprised how effective word-of-mouth (about tooth whitening) can be," says noted author and lecturer William M. Dorfman, DDS, Beverly Hills, CA. "Your patients essentially will be walking spokespeople for your practice. People who are proud of their whiter teeth are sure to share their discovery with friends and family."[26]

QUESTION FOR YOUR NEXT STAFF MEETING
What is it that you and your staff do *so well* that it makes patients want to tell others how good you are?

93 Why patients choose you

A survey of 2687 adults was conducted by the *Wall Street Journal* Online/Harris Interactive Health-Care Poll. Participants were asked which three factors were most important in choosing a doctor and predicting the quality of care one might expect to receive. The results follow[27]:

Factor	Choice	Quality
Physician is part of your insurance plan	46%	n/a
Personal recommendation from someone you know	36%	56%
Physician has a very good reputation	36%	65%
Recommendation or referral from another doctor you trust	35%	57%

Factor	Choice	Quality
The office staff are friendly, helpful, and efficient	27%	49%
Physician's office is in a good location	19%	n/a
Physician has been highly rated in published evaluations of doctors	8%	20%
Physician's patients include many successful and knowledgeable people	3%	6%
Physician has an attractive office in a good building	n/a	3%
Have not chosen a doctor for several years	21%	n/a
None of these	n/a	2%
Not sure/No opinion	n/a	4%

© 2003 American Medical Association

The survey concludes, "Reputation and recommendation were two of the main factors Americans depend on when choosing a physician or predicting a physician's quality of service."

94 Hard-learned lessons about patients' expectations

Richard Boone, a McLean, VA, attorney who defends doctors in malpractice cases, tells me that the common denominator in every lawsuit with which he's been involved has been "failed expectations."

The obvious secret of exceeding patients' expectations: underpromise and over-deliver.

Most patient complaints stem from poorly managed expectations. Don't waste time trying to exceed patient expectations if you and your staff don't have a foolproof system for the basics: delivering *what* you promise, *when* you promise. Make it an unforgivable sin in your practice to make promises that you don't keep.

Consultant Murray Raphel uses the palindromic acronym **D.W.Y.P.Y.W.D.**, which means the same read backwards as forwards: Do What You Promised You Would Do.[28]

"Our premise is simple," says Elizabeth Spaulding, vice president of customer satisfaction, L. L. Bean Inc., "If a product doesn't meet a customer's expectations, whatever they may be, we will replace it, repair it, or refund the customer's money. The point is, the customer determines the expectation. Not us."[29]

"Customers don't care how valuable they are to you. They only care how valuable you are to them" (marketing consultant Don Peppers).

"There is a special feeling that washes over most people when they interact with another human being to whom they are handing money. That feeling is entitlement. They want to be served. They think they *deserve* it."[30]

"In southern California where computer discount stores hang on to solvency by slashing costs and getting by on the flimsiest of margins," says Eric Anderson, MD, San Diego, CA, "a company called ComputerLand Technology Resources flourishes despite its higher prices. A plaque on the wall, displayed where every employee can read it, carries the corporate motto. It says, in part:

We believe business will continue to go where it is invited and remain where it is appreciated.

We believe reputations will continue to be made by many acts and lost by one.

We believe trust, not tricks, will keep clients loyal.

We believe the extra mile has no traffic jams."[31]

95 It starts at the top

Marvin Bower, former director of McKinsey & Company and considered the father of management consulting, has written that it's a manager's responsibility to spell out for employees "the way we do things around here." Bower's implied assumption is that unless you tell people what you want them to do and how you want them to do it, you have no right to expect them to infer by some mysterious means just what you have in mind.[32]

The following letter, sent to a new employee by Peter H. Clayborn, MD, Oak Park, IL, illustrates Bower's principle.

Dear Chris,

Welcome aboard! We are pleased to welcome you to our healthcare team and want you to be part of our continued success. To that end, I want to take a minute to reiterate the reason for our being here. If you remember these principles, I guarantee that you will succeed at your job and reap the rewards. Remember:

Above all, you are here to serve patients. Each of us is. The patient signs our paycheck.

Our practice is built on medical quality and patient service. Strive for uncompromising quality in every phase of your job. Efficiency, precision, and attention to detail are all part of serving the patient.

Every person who walks through our door—patient, postman, management consultant, sales representative—is an honored guest. Each of us is an ambassador of goodwill. We want you to astonish them with your courtesy, concern, and genuine caring for their comfort and well-being.

Know your patients. Greet them by name and with a smile as soon as they walk through our door. Let them know you appreciate them.

Handle any patient problems or complaints with the utmost courtesy, concern, and respect. Remember, the patient is our boss.

In short, we're all working for the same goals. If we apply these principles of patient satisfaction and professional excellence to our particular skills every day, there's no stopping us.

Again, I welcome you to our office and look forward to working with you for a long and rewarding future.

Sincerely,

"When your staff can answer for you based on their deep belief that they know what you stand for," says Irwin M. Becker, DDS, "then they consider themselves your associate. They are not only taking the responsibility of their task, they take on your vision."[33]

REALITY CHECK

"Clarifying the value system and breathing life into it are the greatest contributions a leader can make, say Tom Peters and Robert Waterman in their classic management book *In Search of Excellence*.[34]

Notes

1. McCauley L. How May I Help You, *Fast Company,* March 2000, 93-126.
2. Schlossberg M. Malpractice Reform, *AGD Impact,* July 2003.
3. McCann D. Satisfaction Not Guaranteed, *Dental Practice Report,* July/August 2001, 31-34.
4. King DG. Spa Dentistry. Is it Going Mainstream? *Woman Dentist Journal,* January 2004, 8-12.
5. Jones KC. Consumer Satisfaction: A Key to Financial Success in the Managed Care Environment, *Journal of Health Care Finance,* Summer 1997, 21.
6. Most Important Factor in Service, *Yankelovich Monitor,* 1997, Table 17.25.
7. Wood N. So You Want a Revolution, *Incentive,* June 1998, 41-47.
8. http:www.northshorelij.com.
9. Albrecht K, Bradford LJ. *The Service Advantage,* Dow Jones-Irwin, 1990.
10. Columbo G. Setting and Managing Your Customers' Expectations. *Customer Relationship Management,* November 2003, 32-36.
11. The Importance of the Pre-Clinical Interview. *Dental Practice Advisor,* March 2000, 5.
12. Klokkevold P, Perri G. Incorporating Implants into a Periodontal Practice. *AAP News,* March/April 1998, 9-10.
13. Pelehach L. Crown and Bridge Collection Secrets Revealed. *Dental Practice Report,* March 2003, 54.
14. Lynch S. Helping Manage Patient Expectations. *Dental Economics,* March 2004, 86.
15. Homoly P. How to Profit from Implants. *Dental Economics,* November 1997, 32-36.
16. An Interview with Dr. Larry Rosenthal. *Dental Products Report,* February 1998, 78-86.
17. Q & A With Dr. Wynn Okuda, *Dental Equipment & Materials,* May/June 2003, 81-82.
18. Reichheld FF. The One Number You Need to Grow. *Harvard Business Review,* December 2003, 46-54.
19. Robinette S, Brand C, Lenz V. *Emotion Marketing.* New York: McGraw-Hill, 2001.
20. Henry K. Working Together Through the Years. *Dental Equipment & Materials,* January/February 2004, 59.
21. Fein EB. To Compete, Hospitals Get Hoteliers' Service Lessons. *The New York Times,* July 24, 1995, B1, B6.
22. Kornfeld B. *pm news,* February 12, 2004, issue # 1908, http://www.podiatrym.com.
23. An Interview With Dr. Larry Rosenthal, *Dental Products Report,* February 1998, 78-86.
24. Keller E, Berry J. *The Influentials.* New York: The Free Press, 2003.
25. Taylor J. Word of Mouth Is Where It's At. www.Brandweek,com, June 2, 2003.
26. Dorfman WM. Beaming the News. *Dental Economics,* April 1997, 62-66.
27. amednews.com. Why a Patient Comes to You—and Comes Back. September 15, 2003.

28. Raphel M, Raphel N. *Up The Loyalty Ladder*. New York: HarperBusiness, 1995.
29. McCauley L. How May I Help You? *Fast Company*, March 2000.
30. Steinhauer J. Would a Clerk by Any Other Name Measure Your Feet? *The New York Times*, March 30, 1997.
31. Anderson E. We Need to Get Better at "Customer Service." *Medical Economics*, April 1999, 275-276.
32. Bower M. *The Will to Manage*. NewYork, McGraw-Hill, 1996.
33. Becker I. Building a Five-Star Practice. *California Dental Association Journal*, April, 1995.
34. Peters T, Waterman RJ, Jr. *In Search of Excellence*. New York, Harper & Row, 1982.

8

Secrets of Successful Case Presentations

"Today's smarter, tougher, more cynical, more demanding customer," says *Fortune* magazine, "has less patience than ever for the hard sell—and more opportunity to take his or her business elsewhere."[1]

REALITY CHECK
Forget high-pressure, slick case presentations.

96 The missing ingredient

Did you ever have an "Ah-ha!" moment? One of those times when suddenly everything came together and made perfect sense, and the idea is so basic that you wonder why you didn't see it before?

Mine came when I read that Morton Salt, the world's leading producer of salt, conducted focus groups to learn why its customers were willing to pay a little more for its salt, even though it is identical to all other salt. The company admitted to the participants that its salt was *identical* to that of its competitors, and that it even supplied salt to others who sold it for a lower price.

The group members responded they would *still* buy Morton's salt at the higher price because they *trusted* the company more than others to provide a fair measure and a clean, uncontaminated product.[2]

In other words, *trust* accounts for the loyalty of Morton Salt's customers, not to mention their willingness to pay a premium fee.

REALITY CHECK

Patients don't accept your recommendations for implants, crowns, periodontal surgery, orthodontics, and endodontics because they truly understand the fine points of what's involved. They do so because, in a word, they *trust* you.

97 Put patients' interests first

Trust is the rock-bottom principle on which patient acceptance of your recommendations is based.

"Trust starts with authenticity," say Chip R. Bell and Bilijack R. Bell in *Magnetic Service*. "We trust one another when we perceive his or her motives are genuine or credible. Trust emanates from communication that contains crystal clear content as well as empathetic 'I care about you' consideration. Trust comes from a track record of promises made, paralleled with promises kept. Trust emerges as a result of demonstrated competence that leaves people assured they are dealing with someone with the capacity to perform."[3]

Among all the reasons to put patients' interests first, none are more clinically significant than referring cases beyond your competence and comfort levels.

FROM THE SUCCESS FILES

Dr. Lyle R. Jackson, a veterinarian in Salt Lake City, UT, expressed it well when he told me, "No veterinarian can have all the skills and equipment to do everything. If we perform a procedure, it's because we can do it as well or better than any veterinarian in the Salt Lake City area. If not, we refer the client and say, 'For this procedure, there's another doctor who can do it better. That's not in our best interest, but it's in yours. And that's what matters most.'"

Some practitioners fear that patients will think less of them if they refer a difficult case to a more qualified colleague, when just the opposite happens. Surveys show that patients admire and appreciate doctors who willingly refer special procedures and forgo revenue in the process.

By the same token, patients don't expect a dentist to be good at everything. When you admit your limitations, you *gain* rather than lose stature in your patients' eyes. Your honesty makes you more human and credible and, as Dr. Jackson also noted, it reduces your malpractice risks.

HARD-LEARNED LESSON
The more you act selflessly and put patients' interests first, even when they may be contrary to your own interests, the more trust and patient loyalty you will earn.

Forgo short-term revenue for long-term trust.

98 Anticipate patients' needs

"Anticipating your patients' needs fosters trust," says consultant MaryBeth Head. "It makes them feel you understand. It provides a needed connection that gets your relationship off the ground and keeps it on track. A comfortable, trusting relationship helps patients relax and be receptive. They also will be more at ease asking questions and sharing with you and your staff. Ultimately, this can make the difference in their willingness to accept your findings and treatment recommendations."[4]

ACTION STEP
With your staff, identify those needs patients might have before, during, and after an appointment, and then ask questions designed to meet these needs. The questions might be as simple as asking if they would like to first visit the restroom before starting a lengthy procedure, or asking if the noise of high-speed equipment bothers them and, if it does, providing headphones to listen to music of their choice. The gestures alone will be appreciated.

98 Do one thing great

Trust is built on the belief that you have a higher than normal level of expertise in a specific area. This trust results in greater patient confidence and less "price" sensitivity, as illustrated by the Morton Salt story.

"A person's trust in your expertise is dramatically increased when you focus on doing one thing better than anyone else," says marketing consultant Doug Hall. "When you attempt to be all things to all people, you are perceived as a master of nothing."

"Think hard," Mr. Hall says, "about your offering. "What is the one element that above all others, defines why someone should become your patient? What is the one meaningful difference that is most meaningful to your patients? When your offering is focused, your word of mouth advertising is turbocharged."[5]

FROM THE SUCCESS FILES

"Our office signature," says periodontist Sunie Marchbanks, DDS, Dallas, TX, is periodontal plastic surgery, including gingival grafting and aesthetic crown-lengthening."[6]

100 The role of technology

"I incorporate technology and equipment advances in every patient visit," says Matt Bynum, DDS, Simpsonville, SC. "From the time patients walk in the door, they are visually stimulated with what is new and technologically innovative: from the radio headsets my team and I use to communicate around the office, to the 42 inch plasma screens in every operatory and consultation room, to the 'wireless' radiography we use clinically. Every room is equipped with a computer and flat-screen monitors for patient convenience and easy checkout. Aesthetic cases demand modernization in technique and material."

"Because of the patient's perception of technology and modernization," Dr. Bynum says, "the selling of cases is virtually free of discussion."[7]

101   Hard-learned lessons about trust

Trust is most easily earned through a referral by a patient or, better yet, by a referral from a dental colleague or physician. Patient acceptance at that point is almost a given.

"The patient's first visit is important," says Ken A. Neuman, DMD, FAGD, FACD, FICD, Vancouver, BC. "At this time, we must establish rapport, a sense of trust, and a feeling that the patient has made the correct decision in selecting our office to entrust with the care of his mouth."[8]

There's little doubt that most dentists can look into the mouth of almost any new patient and find treatable problems. Pointing out all those problems on a patient's *first visit* would for many, however, be going too fast, too soon—especially if it's the first time the patient is hearing about them.

"Be very slow to get into the patient's mouth," says periodontist Mitchell T. Cantor, DMD, MSD. "First, get into the patient's *heart*; then, the patients *head*; and *then*, into the patient's mouth."

"What dentistry doesn't get done this year," says consultant Paul Homoly, DDS, "you'll do next year. Think long term and you'll prosper."[9]

"The primary differentiating factor in treatment acceptance rates among practices is one of trust," says the *Blair/McGill Advisory*. "Trust by the patient is based upon the belief that the doctor and staff care for the patient as an individual, and for their well being, not merely as someone with dollars to spend that can help the doctor reach his or her financial goals. This belief is typically based on the quality of care provided by the doctor and staff."[10]

"Trust has become so scarce a commodity," observed Harold Wirth, DDS, "that any dentist who earns a reputation for caring and being trustworthy will quickly acquire as many patients as he can handle. Why? Because people still cherish the values that seem to have been lost and are overjoyed to learn that care and trust still exist."[11]

"We go overboard to try to take care of patients' needs," says Dave Smith, DDS, Fishers, IN. "We earn our patients' trust and respect by going beyond the call of duty." "That commitment," writes Barbara Baccei, "is evidenced by the doctors' willingness to respond personally to emergencies, make follow-up calls after difficult treatments, and invest in the people, systems, and facilities that have totally transformed the way the community of Fishers, Indiana looks at dentistry."[12]

"If all dentists acted like *they assumed patients trusted them* and would take their advice," says periodontist Douglas M. Neuman, DMD, Lexington, KY, "then all they would need to do is decide in their own mind what treatment is necessary—be it grafts, crown-lengthening, pocket surgery, crowns, bridges, implants, etc.—and then *tell their patients exactly that.*"[13]

102 Maintain patient confidentiality

'There is no faster way to build a foundation of trust," says consultant Susan Keane Baker, "than to be absolutely fanatical about patient confidentiality. Letting a patient know you are committed to patient confidentiality will cement your relationship faster than almost anything else you can do."[14]

ACTION STEP

Requiring staff members to sign confidentiality agreements on an annual basis is a good way to maintain awareness of the importance of protecting patients' privacy.

FROM THE SUCCESS FILES

The following item appeared in a patient newsletter from the office of Albert Ousborne, DDS, Thomas Keller, DDS, and Patrick Ousborne, DDS, Towson, MD.

"Drs. Ousborne and Keller sponsored an educational course which was also attended by many of our invited dental colleagues in the community. This course, taught by Chris Wisnon, a Nurse Educator at The University of Maryland Dental School, provided us with the latest information on confidentiality and protecting the privacy of our patients. Drs. Ousborne and Keller have always been careful to maintain confidentiality. Now we will take even greater measures to further elevate our standard of care to meet the new federal HIPPA requirements."[15]

103 Self-confidence

Self-confidence is one of the qualities that inspires trust in others. Dentists who have it radiate a reassuring sense that they know what they're doing.

Earl Nightingale, who in his time was the most listened-to-radio broadcaster on earth, tried to define this quality that is common to top performers in all fields. "To begin," he said, "they are in work which comes close to perfectly matching their natural talents; they are not just round pegs in round holes; rather they are uniquely shaped pegs which have found perfectly matching, uniquely shaped holes. When they are doing that at which they excel, they are in their element and are happier than anywhere else."

"They also know they are good," Nightingale said, "have supreme confidence in themselves and develop what I call a 'consciousness of competence.' This is what causes them to relax to the degree necessary for greatness in anything. While others are nervously straining to excel, forcing themselves and in this forcing, falling short, the stars are relaxed in the knowledge of their own greatness. They don't always win, but over the years this attitude keeps them in the elite ranks of stardom."[16]

REALITY CHECK

One of the reasons that dentists attending intensive, hands-on, post-graduate programs throughout the country are so successful is they leave these programs with confidence in their abilities. "Patients are perceptive," says Gary M. Radz, DDS, Denver, CO. "They know when we are certain in our abilities—and when we aren't."[17]

HARD-LEARNED LESSON

They key to success, says business visionary/author Peter Drucker, is to discover what you're good at, and then become exceptional at it. "And it's amazing," he adds, "how few people know what they're good at."[18]

104 Walk your talk

"It was one of the best investment decisions of my career," says Stephen C. Brown, DDS, Richmond, VA. "I had eight veneers placed to close some rather large diastemas, and the effect has been tremendous. Not only has it improved my self-esteem and appearance, but it has helped my dental practice as well. I now find that case presentations are much more likely to be accepted than they were before. (I'm doing at least five times the number of veneer cases as I was before treatment.)"

"After explaining what veneers can do for one's appearance, I smile and show the patient what mine look like. This gives the treatment instant credibility."[19]

ACTION STEP

"If you have not restored the mouths of your staff and yourself, " says Stephen D. Poss, DDS, Smyrna, TN, "do it now! It is hard for your staff members to be missionaries for your practice by suggesting inlays and veneers when they have wall-to-wall amalgams, as well as stained and crowded front teeth."

"We took one summer and spent several Friday mornings," Dr. Poss says, "and made it mandatory for my staff members to have their mouths ideally restored. If they are good, long-term employees, do it for free or just the lab fee. As a result, they will sell more dentistry than you can imagine."[20]

HARD-LEARNED LESSON

"If a dentist is trying to practice appearance-related dentistry and has an ugly smile," says David S. Hornbrook, DDS, FAACD, San Diego, CA, "it is not going to work."[21]

105 Explain the pros and cons

Patients tend to be impressed with and have more trust in dentists who explain both the pros and cons of treatment alternatives. Doing so imbues the dentist's recommendations with a sense of balance and honesty, and makes them more believable.

FROM THE SUCCESS FILES

"I place a great deal of emphasis on explaining to patients what I recommend for them, and why," says Gerard R. Valentini, DDS, Delray Beach, FL. "This builds trust and increases patients' comfort level. They are more relaxed."

"Like all dentists, after I've diagnosed a problem—whether it be periodontal disease, a cracked tooth, or a denture that no longer fits properly, I may be aware of several treatment options. So I take the time to explain why a particular treatment option is best for that patient at that time. If more than one option is suitable, I explain the advantages and disadvantages of each. This way, patients understand that my recommendations are not based on how much money I might make or other self-serving reasons, but on what is in each patient's best interest. This also helps build patient trust."[22]

REALITY CHECK

Extensive research shows that two-sided messages, presenting both advantages and disadvantages, are judged more trustworthy than messages that present only one-sided messages, says Daniel J. O'Keefe in *Persuasion: Theory and Research,* 2nd edition.

106 Make the patient a co-diagnostician

"The intraoral video examination," says Ronald E. Goldstein, DDS, Atlanta, GA, "is an effective means of establishing trust between patient and dentist by making the patient a co-diagnostician. In fact, it is not uncommon for patients to stop the diagnosis and ask specific questions about what they see. In this way, patients can begin to diagnose pathology even before the dentist mentions it. A major benefit of the video examination to the dentist is that invariably the examination reveals conditions not seen in typical clinical examinations—even when using magnification loupes."[23]

ACTION STEP

Transform your patient from a passive entity to an active diagnostician engaged in the exam, says consultant Amy Morgan, CEO of the Pride Institute. "Explain the meaning of the periodontal probings and ask the patient to track readings of four or higher as you call them out. During the dentition exam, explain the significance of missing tooth structure and then ask your patient to keep track of those teeth having greater than half of their tooth structure missing, as they may need more permanent restorations. This is done while you call out the percentage of missing tooth to an assistant."[24]

REALITY CHECK

"When patients can visualize the actual condition of their own mouth," says Phillip Bonner, DDS, Editor-in-Chief of *Dentistry Today*, "it is easy to understand why the dentist is recommending specific treatments. They suddenly 'own' their problem and want a solution. They become active participants in the diagnostic process and their individual treatment plan."[25]

107 Be low-key

"I take great pride and satisfaction in telling a patient, 'I didn't find anything that needs to be treated at this time,'" says Joe Steven Jr., DDS, Wichita, KS. "I even break the Great Gurus' Golden Rule and will actually *watch* suspicious areas. Patients love you for this conservative approach and that's one of the things that help generate new-patient referrals. They're proud to recommend you to their friends and family because they trust you and know their friends will be treated properly."[26]

FROM THE SUCCESS FILES

Dr. Gordon Christensen has said that bleaching teeth is perhaps the most behavior-changing procedure in dentistry. He adds that when patients have their teeth bleached, they often become interested in veneers, replacements of old restorations, diastema closures, and other aesthetic procedures.

"Our philosophy in our approach to patient care is to always be as conservative as possible," says Lou Graham, DDS, Chairperson of the University of Chicago Dental School's Department of Surgery and who maintains a large group practice with 5 locations throughout Chicago. "This can translate into orthodontics versus veneers, early laser caries detection, pulp-capping symptom-free teeth with carious exposures, and non-surgical periodontal therapies. This does not mean we do not do veneer smiles; but if patients wish to undergo orthodontics and have beautiful, natural teeth afterwards, this is ultimately the most conservative long-term treatment possible. Obviously, many combinations of treatment may be needed, which only reinforces the importance of understanding the individual needs of your patient. Thus, the keys to that first visit are listening, sharing, and offering a variety of treatments best-suited for that particular patient."[27]

ACTION STEP

William Dorfman, DDS, Beverly Hills, CA, recommends an easy, low-key approach to introduce the subject of bleaching. After examining the patient, he says, the dentists should simply look the person in the eye and ask, "Would you like whiter teeth?" Most people, he reports, say "yes."

If you're not comfortable doing that, says Dr. Dorfman, have your hygienist ask the question at the conclusion of the prophylaxis, or to be even lower key, include it on the health history form.[28]

108 Learn what matters to patients

"Trust emerges when a patient feels cared about as a person," says Charles L. Milone, DDS, "when the patient believes you are sensitive and caring, and when the patient senses you are trying to understand his or her feelings."[29]

During the interview, listen to and observe the patient closely," says Justin Lee Altshuler, DMD, FICD, clinical professor at Boston University's Goldman School of Dental Medicine. "What does the patient's body language tell you? Does the patient seem relaxed, anxious, hurried, or stressed? What kind of previous experiences has the patient had with dentistry? What was the patient's last dental treatment, and was it completed? Are there any dental issues that the patient feels are a top priority? Are there any dental treatments that the patient is curious about, but may not consider critical? By gleaning answers to these questions, you can begin to make educated decisions about how receptive the patient will be to your treatment recommendations, including recommendations for elective procedures."[30]

HARD-LEARNED LESSON

Five major roadblocks exist to case acceptance: No need, no trust, no interest, no hurry, and no ability to pay or decide on one's own. The challenge is to identify which if any of these problems causes a patient to decline or delay treatment. Responding to the wrong problem, no matter how brilliantly, just isn't going to work.

109 Ask need-clarifying questions

Many dentists believe that talking is more important than listening, but using questions is the only way you can find out what's on a patient's mind. Through questions you can determine a patient's expectations, perceived needs, priorities, and concerns, and it's essential that you learn these things if your case presentations are to be on target.

One example of a need-clarifying question is "What concerns, if any, do you have about today's visit?"

FROM THE SUCCESS FILES

"Pay particular attention to your patient's concerns," says Larry Rosenthal, DDS, New York, NY. "Ask more questions: 'Tell me more about that' will always get a response. How do they feel about time: is it an issue? How do they feel about pain: is fear an issue? Never assume you know what a patient is going to tell you. Always keep asking patients about their concerns. Always keep asking questions and gathering information. Then you can address those concerns strongly. Do not, under any circumstances, avoid them."[31]

"On a scale of 1 to 10 (1 being low and 10 being high) what priority do you give your teeth?"

Such a question enables you to learn your patient's perceived needs and, with follow-up questions, why they feel that way. You'll then have a chance to upgrade the thinking of those with low-priority answers.

"Have dental procedures ever been recommended to you that you didn't have done?"

If the answer to this question is "yes," it's logical to try to learn what the patient's objection was before recommending the same procedure and encountering the same problem.

FROM THE SUCCESS FILES

"The initial forms can provide a plethora of knowledge for the dentist as he or she meets the patient for the first time," says Lou Graham, DDS, Chicago, IL. "Questions asked on our forms include the following:

Are you happy with your smile?

If not, what would you like to improve?

Do you want to keep your teeth throughout your lifetime?"

"These questions," says Dr. Graham, "allow the dentist to gain an understanding of the patient's interest in aesthetic dentistry and to determine how important it is to them to preserve their dentition. Even if patients are happy with their smiles, the dentist can still review the correctness of occlusion and the color of the teeth, as well as discuss various oral-health needs. It is critical that the initial appointment *not* be a sales appointment (as too many are) but one in which the patient and the doctor establish a relationship with each other. This one point is the key to success for many practitioners and the reason for failure for others."[32]

HARD-LEARNED LESSON

"The simple act of asking questions and then deeply listening to the patient's responses," says Ron Schefdore, DMD, Burr Ridge, IL, "has made the single greatest difference in my practice and the way our patents experience our practice."[33]

110 Engage patients' self-interest

Instead of *telling* patients about the aesthetic imperfections you see, engage their self-interest by *asking* patients about them. For example, you can ask the patient the following questions:

"Does this space between your front teeth bother you?"

"Have you ever noticed this bottom tooth is tilted over more than any of the others in your mouth?"

Similar questions can be asked of patients with chipped, missing, broken, discolored, misshaped, or excessively worn teeth.

Dentists tell me that a surprising number of patients have never noticed or thought about such matters until they were pointed out. Other patients were aware of these conditions but never realized anything could be done about them. An intraoral video camera or hand mirror, an explanation of how these problems can be corrected, before-and-after photos of previous cases, or an actual demonstration of what can be done often arouse self-motivation and produce immediate patient acceptance.

FROM THE SUCCESS FILES

"Ask questions that cause clients to think," says author Mary Osborne, RDH, Seattle, WA. "Many people go on automatic pilot when they go to a dentist. They don't expect to be asked to participate, so they don't plan to take an active part in the visit. If either "yes" or "no" can answer all the questions you pose, there is not much thinking involved for them. Open-end questions are more likely to engage patients."

"Instead of asking if there have been any changes in the health history," Ms. Osborne says, "try asking, 'What changes have you noticed in your health since I saw you last?' Instead of asking if they have to decided to go ahead with the treatment you've recommended, try asking, 'What have you been thinking about the bridge we talked about last time?'"[34]

111 Seeing is believing

In his book *Winning the Interaction Game*, Ralph Laurie writes, "A University of Minnesota study showed the use of visual aids in a presentation increased the likelihood of a successful outcome by 43 percent. Furthermore, the study uncovered that people were willing to pay 26 percent more for the same product after visual aids were incorporated into the presentation about the product. A similar study conducted at the Wharton School of Business found that visual aids reduced the time required to explain complex procedures by 25 to 40 percent."[35]

"We now have an array of digital imaging and photography technologies at our disposal," says Phillip Bonner, DDS, "and dentists are discovering how powerful these tools can be for educating patients about dental health, as well as dramatically increasing patient acceptance."[36]

"High-resolution, large-format, digital-radiographic images, for example, optimized to display what you want to show," says David Gane, DDS, vice president of PracticeWorks, Inc., "are easy for patients to understand. Displaying the images on a large monitor also helps to optimize communication. This type of visual communication increases education and trust, leading ultimately to patient agreement. Patient agreement leads to increased treatment acceptance which in turn, leads to increased revenue."[37]

FROM THE SUCCESS FILES

"Any cosmetic or restorative dentist and any orthodontist desiring to increase case acceptance—whether it be for cosmetic, anterior, functional, or full-mouth treatment—can utilize and benefit from the cosmetic-imaging process," says David J. Sultanov, DMD, Pittsburgh, PA.

"Patients cannot easily visualize comfortable, functioning dentistry with healthy periodontal tissues, but cosmetic imaging's ability to show them their enhanced appearance after treatment could be the primary reason they choose a dental procedure. There's an emotional impact in seeing yourself with a greatly improved smile," Dr. Sultanov says.

"Computer imaging," he adds, "projects your practice as a high-tech operation. Even if patients are not interested in aesthetics, they leave their appointment feeling that you are on the cutting edge of dentistry."[38]

REALITY CHECK

A cosmetic-imaging system can also determine whether a patient's demands and expectations are realistic or beyond your ability to meet.

---

112 Don't prejudge patients

"Keep in mind while you do your examination," says Joseph Graskemper, DDS, JD, Bellport, NY, "not to prejudge a patient as to what he or she would like to have done. Make your treatment plan to be the ideal. It's easier to change a treatment plan during treatment to a less costly alternative, than to change to a more expensive option."[39]

ACTION STEP

Make *clinical* decisions for patients, not *economic* decisions. Recommend what's best for patients, and let them decide if that's what they want.

FROM THE SUCCESS FILES

"I used to assume that patients only wanted traditional restorations," says Tony Ratliff, DDS, MBA, Fishers, IN. "I have found it best not to assume, but to educate, motivate, and ask. A few more inlays a week, an additional six veneers, or two extra bleaching procedures will have a dramatic effect on your bottom line. These additional elective cosmetic services or 'upgraded' restorations will have a cumulative effect over the course of a month or even a year. After adopting an "educated motivation" philosophy, I think you will be amazed at the number of patients who will choose elective cosmetic services when given the option."[40]

HARD-LEARNED LESSON

"Of all the factors that should influence a dentist's selection of restorative materials," says Michael C. DiTolla, DDS, FAGD, Downey, CA, "the only one that the dentist has no business deciding and is completely unqualified to make, is the cost factor. Yet, cost was the very reason why nearly all patients have mouths full of amalgam and weren't given the option of superior material. The dentist's role is to offer the restorations and materials that fit the parameters of the clinical situation, while the patient's role is to choose a restoration from those suggested by the dentist that fits his or her aesthetic, financial, and longevity priorities."[41]

113 Timing is everything

"Our biggest fault in treatment presentation," say Phil Korpi, DDS, and Scott Henricksen, DDS, Seattle, WA, "is in discussing treatment prematurely, before the patient has grasped that he indeed has periodontal disease that needs treatment. Therefore don't use visual aids or drawings" they advise, "that depict treatment when you are discussing the progression of periodontal disease. Be sure your drawings and visual aids show disease progression only, until the patient asks about treatment. Then use a separate visual aid for that."[42]

114 Make dentistry affordable

"If you want to increase case acceptance," says Louis Malcmacher, DDS, Bay Village, OH, "offer third party financing to every patient who walks through the door. When you tell a patient that a treatment plan that totals $3000 will cost him or her only $70 per month for 42 months, it communicates that the treatment really can be worked into their budgets."

"Part of my treatment presentation," Dr. Malcmacher says, "is to reassure patients we will work with them to make treatment affordable. By the time my office manager and I are finished with a case presentation, patients know we are on their side and are relieved to discover they really can afford the best dental treatment possible."[43]

ɔy offering nonrecourse outside financing as the first and preferred method of paying for treatment," says consultant/speaker Debra Engelhardt Nash, "a higher patient acceptance level will be achieved."

In this way, "patients can proceed with their treatment of choice, and the fee has been comfortably budgeted for them. The practice receives full payment within days of submitting the treatment fee and removes the liability of carrying patient balances."

"Lending companies do receive a percentage of the treatment fee in remuneration for their services," Ms. Nash says, "depending on the amount borrowed and the credit rating of the applicant. Some offices balk at this charge without realizing what the office is saving in time and resources. First, statements do not have to be sent to the patient. Also, the staff does not have to monitor the account, make collection calls, personally turn patients over to collections services, or track third-party payments."[44]

ACTION STEP

"Begin communicating with your patient base," suggests consultant/speaker Sally McKensie, "especially those patients to whom you have extended credit and who are still paying monthly. You may want to send them a letter and convert their payment plan to the third-party financing company. Then, go through your files and identify patients who may have declined or delayed treatment due to financial concerns."[45]

115 Make it easy for patients to say "yes"

The final phase of a treatment conference is the "close." It's the point at which the patient is asked to make a commitment to proceed with treatment. It's also the most critical part of the conference, because nothing really happens in dentistry until the patient says "yes."

The problem for many dentists is that they're poor "closers." As a result, more patients than necessary leave without making a decision, saying they want to think it over, talk to their spouse, or perhaps seek another opinion. There are several reasons for this all-too-common failure to close.

One problem is the tendency to tell patients too much, which results in "information overload," confusion, or indecision.

Another problem is the tremendous inertia people have about making healthcare decisions, especially about elective procedures that involve pain, a large block of time, and high out-of-pocket costs. They'd rather ignore the problem, hope for the best, and procrastinate for as long as possible.

A principal reason why many dentists hesitate to close is their belief that closing is in some way underhanded and manipulative.

REALITY CHECK

Closing isn't pressuring people into treatment they don't need. Rather, it's helping patients to overcome inertia and make decisions that are in their best interests. In fact, failing to close could be viewed as a *disservice* to the patient.

One of the best ways to bring a case presentation to a close is with the sentence "Where do we go from here?" This question, used when all needs have been identified and all solutions are explained, can help the patient feel comfortable enough to proceed with the treatment plan.

POSITIVE ACTION QUESTIONS

"Positive action questions," says author/speaker Nate Booth, DDS, "encourage patients to take numerous small steps to case acceptance, rather than one big commitment at the end. Most people prefer to take small steps, so it's best to sprinkle these questions throughout your case presentations. An example of a positive action question is 'Does Option A or B look better to you?'"[46]

TRIAL CLOSE QUESTIONS

The next step in asking patients for a commitment is what's called a "trial close." It's basically a check on how the patient is reacting to what you have said. For example, following your recommendations, ask any of the following low-key questions:

"How does this sound so far?"

"Does that make sense?"

"Are there any other concerns that need to be resolved?"

Regardless of how the patient answers, you'll know where you and the patient stand. A prolonged pause or an ambivalent response may indicate the need for more discussion, perhaps with a staff member if a financial issue is involved. If you've done a good job, the patient will have no questions and may be ready to proceed.

ACTION CLOSE QUESTIONS

The next step is called the "action close" (also named the "assumptive close" because it assumes the patient is comfortable with your recommendations and ready to proceed). All that may be needed is this simple question:

"Should we schedule an appointment to begin your treatment?"

FROM THE SUCCESS FILES

"If you are looking to increase your profitability in restorative dentistry," says Ted Morgan, DDS, Gotham, ME, "make sure you ask every patient to do the treatment after you have explained your recommendation to them. It's easy! Just say something like, "Does this sound like something you would want to do?"[47]

"During any given day," says speaker Kristine A. Hodsdon, RDH, BS, "you could have just completed a top-notch, comprehensive, prediagnostic clinical analysis with appropriate radiographs, intraoral pictures, educational tools, high-tech gadgets, etc. You have a complete understanding about the client's perspective of his or her oral health needs, wants, concerns, and smile desires. But if you do not ask the final question about getting started, the patient probably will not do it. So make sure you conclude with the statement: 'Would you like to schedule it today?'"[48]

REALITY CHECK

"If patients say 'no' to my best case presentation," says Gary M. Radz, DDS, Denver, CO, "I don't take it personally. 'No' simply means, 'I'm just not ready yet.'"[49]

116 Beware of overkill

The treatment conference is unquestionably the key to helping patients best understand your recommendations. What you want to avoid is *overkill,* which occurs when dentists get carried away with patient education and tell patients *more* than they want to hear or need to know.

Why do some dentists go overboard on case presentation? The reasons include the following:

- They overestimate their patients' interest in learning "everything" about the diagnosis, the etiology of the problem, and the recommendations, and include in the process a complete battery of study models, X-rays, and patient education materials.
- Some believe that the more they explain, the more persuasive they are, and the better the chances that patients will say "yes" to their recommendations.
- Others fail to notice a patient's blank stare while they're talking or other signs that the patient has lost all interest in what they're saying.

In short, the trap into which these well-meaning, overly-talkative dentists fall is thinking more about what they want to *say* than what the patient wants to *hear*.

If you think you may at times be guilty of "overexplaining," here's a strategy that may help. After a minute or two of nonstop talking about the benefits of restorative implant therapy for missing or defective dentition (or whatever the subject) *stop talking* and ask the patient, "Is this interesting?"

If the patient says, "yes," keep going. Even better, if the patient says, "Yes, and you're the first doctor who ever explained this to me," give yourself a pat on the back, and keep talking. You've hit a home run.

But if the patient replies to your question with only a shrug and a look of little interest in hearing more about the subject, cut your explanation short. You'll save time, prevent overkill, and have a happier patient.

FROM THE SUCCESS FILES

Author/speaker Nate Booth, DDS, suggests this simple question: "Would you like all the details about the treatment that needs to be done, or just an overview?"[50]

REALITY CHECK

"We dentists spend so much time trying to help our patients understand what we are going to do and why this course of treatment is in their best interest that we lose them in the process," says Gary M. Radz, DDS, Denver, CO. "We create confusion—or worse, make our patients feel we are trying to 'sell' them something."[51]

ACTION STEP

To learn if you're possibly more talkative than you intend or need to be, critique yourself. (See Secret #140.)

117 Hard-learned lessons about case presentation

"If you're selling a service," says Harry Beckwith, author of *Selling the Invisible,* "you're selling a relationship."

"Patients don't purchase dentistry," says consultant/speaker James F. Pride, DDS. "Patients purchase aesthetics, function, a friendly and comfortable environment peopled by a dental team with whom they have a pleasant, trusting relationship. This quality combination is not something patients can find in just any dental practice."[52]

"The need to do case presentation well," says Ted Morgan, DDS, Gotham, ME, goes much deeper than profit. It is basic to the fulfillment of our responsibility to our patients, who trust us with their care. Failing to find, understand, and address their real needs whenever possible is failing to give optimal care."[53]

"The worst case presentations I do," says Anthony S. Feck, DMD, Lexington, KY, "are when I do all the talking. When I do that, I don't have a clue as to what really matters to the patient, and no case presentation can be effective until that is decided. The best way to determine that is to ask good questions and listen carefully to the answers."[54]

"The total fee required to restore optimal oral health," says John A. Wilde, DDS, New Albany, IN, "is presented *only* after all needed treatment is fully understood by the patient."[55]

People can't value what they don't understand.

People won't buy what they don't value.

"It's easy to make assumptions about patients' desires based on outward appearances or insurance status," says Stephen D. Poss, DDS, Smyrna, TN. "For example, a 70-year-old local farmer came to my office. He had 10 teeth that were chipped and worn, and requested aesthetic, metal-free dentistry to restore his smile. He specifically explained he did not want the dark 'collars' associated with PFM restorations but rather a natural-looking, aesthetic smile. His appearance suggested he couldn't afford a prophy, much less the aesthetic smile enhancements he requested. By the time he left the office, however, we had decided on a 10-unit IPS Empress2 reconstruction, and he wrote a check for the full amount in advance. Although this case is not the norm, it stands as an important lesson for those who don't believe small-town cosmetic dentists can succeed. It all comes down to language and knowing the right questions to ask."[56]

Don't oversell patients on procedures they don't really want or can afford. They may later experience "buyer's remorse." Dissatisfied with the final result, patients may not follow through with payments, or worse, they may "bad mouth" you to others.

"Get really good at saying, 'When you're ready . . .' says consultant/author Paul Homoly, DDS. "Let people know you're happy to proceed with their care, based on *their* schedule and *their* budget."[57]

"If worse comes to worse," says David C. Steele, DDS, FICD, FAGD, Alexandria, IN, "offer something like, 'If you're unsure, let's do what you want done right now to make you feel like you're heading in the direction you want, then we'll do other treatment if you like.'"[58]

Notes

1. Power C, Driscoll L, Bohn E. Smart Selling: How Companies Are Winning Over Today's Tougher Customer. *Fortune*, August 3, 2002, 47-48.
2. Brainstorming. *Bottom Line/Business*, October 1996, 15.
3. Bell CR, Bell BR. *Magnetic Service*. San Francisco: Berrett-Koehler Publishers, Inc., 2003.
4. Head M. Anticipation: Meeting Your Patient's Fundamental Needs. *Dental Economics*, March 2004, 137-138, 161.
5. Hall D. *Meaningful Marketing*. Cincinnati, OH, Brain Brew Books, 2003.
6. Marchbanks SA. Twist on Pain Reduction. *Woman Dentist Journal*, April 2004, 8, 10-11.
7. Winters K. Case Acceptance Tips. *Dental Equipment & Materials*, March/April 2003, 35.
8. Neuman KA. Maximizing the Use of an Intraoral Camera. *Dentistry Today*, July 2003, 72-75.
9. Homoly P. I'll Go Home and Think about It. *Dental Economics*, August 2002.
10. Increase Treatment Acceptance Through Improved Quality of Care. *Blair/McGill Advisory*, March 2003, 3.
11. Wirth H. The Role of Empathy in a Relationship Based Dental Practice. www.SpiritofCaring.com.
12. Baccei B. How a Building Can 'Really Smile.' *Dental Economics*, April 2000, 64-74.
13. Neuman DM. Some Advice for Dr. New. *Dental Graduate*, May 1999, 6, 76.

14. Baker SK. *Managing Patient Expectations*. San Francisco: Jossey-Bass Publishers, 1998.

15. Ousborne A, Keller T. O/K Hosts Seminar for Dentists and Staff. *Chairside Chatter*, Spring 2003, 3.

16. Nightingale E. *This is Earl Nightingale*. Chicago, IL: Nightingale-Conant Corporation, 1977.

17. Radz GM. It's a Case Presentation—Not Dentistry "101." *Dental Economics*, November 2000, 86-90.

18. Rubin H. Peter's Principles, *Inc*. March 1998, 62-68.

19. Brown SC. Building Confidence and the Bottom Line. *Dental Practice & Finance*, September/October, 1997, 47.

20. Poss SD. Eight Priorities for Establishing Yourself as an Esthetic Dentist—Even in the Boondocks. *Dental Economics*, October 1998, 52-53.

21. An Interview with Dr. David S. Hornbrook. *Dental Products Report*, September 1997, 104-107.

22. Valentini GR. Building Relationships Builds the Practice. *Dentistry Today*, April 2003, 102-104.

23. Goldstein RE. Intraoral Cameras Help Predict and Prevent Tooth Loss. *Contemporary Esthetics and Restorative Practice*, October 2001, 1-2.

24. Morgan A. How to Enjoy and Even Love "Selling" Complete Dentistry, Strategies for Success. Supplement to *Dental Economics*, September 2003.

25. Bonner P. The Power of Co-Diagnosis. *Dentistry Today*, April 2003, 12.

26. Steven J, Jr. "Only the Best Quality Dentistry"... Oh, Really? *Dental Economics*, August 2003, 16-18, 138.

27. Graham L. How to Profit from Whitening. *Dental Economics*, June 2003, 124-126, 157.

28. Dorfman W. Beaming the News. *Dental Economics*, April 1997, 62-66.

29. Milone CL. *Stress Management for the Dental Team*. Philadelphia: Lea & Febiger, 1986.

30. Altshuler JL. Digital Imaging Enhances Whitening Case Acceptance. *Dental Economics*, March 2003, 84-88.

31. Rosenthal L. How to Develop an Esthetic-Centered Practice. *Dental Economics*, January 1997, 26-29.

32. Graham L. Tooth-Whitening Is In. *Dental Economics*, June 2003, 124-126, 157.

33. Schefdore R. Better Service, Better Dentistry, Better Income. *Dentistry Today*, December 2003, 10.

34. Osborne M. Staying in the Question: The most powerful patient communication tool you can use. Part III. http://:www.spiritofcaring.com.

35. Laurie R. *Winning the Interaction Game*, 4th edition. Vancouver, WA: Caesy Education Systems, 2002.

36. Bonner P. The Power of Co-Diagnosis. *Dentistry Today*, April 2003, 12.

37. Gane D. Solid-State Digital Radiography. *Dental Economics*, April 2003, 100-108.

38. Sultanov DJ. Cosmetic Imaging for Profitability. *Dental Economics*, November 2001.

39. Graskemper J. How to Sell a Treatment Plan: Codiagnosing. *Dentistry Today*, October 2000, 41-43.

40. Ratliff T. How to Profit from Cosmetic Dentistry. *Dental Economics,* November 2001.
41. DiTolla MC. Giving Patients Freedom of Choice. *Dental Economics,* February 1998, 10, 12, 87.
42. Korpi P, Henricksen S. Winning the Mind of the Patient: The Missing Link in Periodontal Treatment Acceptance. *Dentistry Today,* February 2001, 92-95.
43. Malcmacher L. Can Your Patients Afford You? *Dental Economics,* March 2004, 60.
44. Nash DE. Discretionary Dentistry. *Contemporary Esthetics and Restorative Practice,* May 1999.
45. Jameson J. Top Management Consultants Speak Out . . . Outsourcing Patient Financing. *Dental Economics,* December 2002.
46. Booth N. Sleuthing for the Right Questions to Ask. *Dental Economics,* April 1999, 54-56.
47. Morgan T. Case Acceptance Is Cornerstone of Dental Wall. *Dental Economics,* February 1998, 28-34, 69.
48. Hodsdon KA. Get Comfortable With Fees. *RDH,* December 2001.
49. Radz GM. It's a Case Presentation—Not "Dentistry 101." *Dental Economics,* November 2000, 86-90.
50. Booth N. Sleuthing for the Right Questions to Ask. *Dental Economics,* April 1999, 54-56.
51. Radz GM. It's a Case Presentation—Not "Dentistry 101." *Dental Economics,* November 2000, 86-90.
52. *Taking Your Practice to a New Level.* St. Paul, MN: 3M Dental Products, 1999.
53. Morgan T. Case Acceptance Is Cornerstone of Dental Wall. *Dental Economics,* February 1998, 28-32, 69.
54. Feck AS. Seven Steps to Increasing Case Acceptance. *Dental Economics,* February 1998, 36-40, 58.
55. Wilde JA. Ask! *Dental Economics,* February 2003, 152-154.
56. Poss SD. How to Profit from Endodontics. *Dental Economics,* November 1999.
57. Homoly P. Dancing With Patients. *Dental Economics,* June 2000, 26.
58. Steele DC. *Optimizing Dental Care: Exceptional Case Presentation.* Tulsa, OK: PennWell Books, 1996.

9

Hard-Learned Lessons About Fees

During a seminar I conducted for accountants, I met a middle-aged practitioner whose specialty was agricultural economics. He told me that several years before, he had suffered a major heart attack, spent close to 2 months in the hospital and then additional time at home before returning to work on a part-time basis. His physician's advice was succinct and no-nonsense: "Cut your work load and client list in half, or you're not going to make it!"

Sensing the life and death consequences of the situation, this hard-working accountant heeded his doctor's advice. He wrote to each of his tax and audit clients explaining the situation, his need to cut back on his practice, and (with an eye on keeping his practice economically afloat) the need to double his fees!

He added that he recognized this would create a hardship for some of his clients and would understand if they needed to transfer their records and future work to another practitioner. He ended the letter by asking his clients to please call his office with further instructions.

How did his clients react to the letter?

More than 90% called to say they would remain with him.

Obviously, a number of factors accounted for this allegiance. But the question remains: How important are fees?

The answer: probably less than you think.

118 Fees are important—but not that important

"Industry research shows that as many as 85 percent of service station customers are not loyal," say consultants Jill Griffin and Michael W. Lowenstein, authors of *Customer WinBack*. "Mobil Oil wanted to know why. The company conducted its own market research among over two thousand motorists and found only 20 percent buy strictly on price. Although wanting competitive pricing, most buyers also desired things like more human contact, fast service, clean restrooms, ease of getting in and out of the facility, and attendants who recognize them. So Mobil went to work to improve its stations with better lighting and cleaner facilities and attendant friendliness and responsiveness. The company's initiatives were rewarded with revenues increasing by 15 to 20 percent at many of their stations."[1]

Studies of consumer behavior indicate that, on average, only 13% of people make buying decisions based *strictly* on price. The consumers in this small group, either because of economic circumstances or because they don't know better, always look for the lowest price. That means 87% of people consider price but *also* look for quality care, service, convenience, a personal relationship, and more from their service providers.

Considering the buying potential of each group, does it make sense to gear your practice and fee structure to the price-conscious 13% of the population? You may drown in overhead costs trying to keep prices low enough to suit them, and by definition, they will leave your practice if they can find lower fees elsewhere.

You may be thinking that more than 13% of your community is price-conscious. Perhaps this is true, but even if you double this number, that leaves 74% of people who are interested in factors other than cost—still a sizable target population for your practice. If you tripled the figure to 39 percent, you could still target 61 percent of the population as prospective patients—more than you and your present staff could handle.

You can't be all things to all people, so why not provide the quality of care, personal service, convenience, and one-to-one relationships that meet the needs of the 87% to whom price isn't everything?

REALITY CHECK

If price were everything, supermarket shelves would be filled with generic products priced lower than their branded counterparts. As it is, generic products account for only a small fraction of supermarket sales.

---

119 Perceived value

"A fair fee," as L.D. Pankey, DDS, defines it, "is that fee which the patient is willing to pay and the doctor is willing to receive—with gratitude."

Picture a balance scale. If in the patient's mind, the *fee* outweighs the *perceived value* of your treatment plan, he or she may want to "think about it," perhaps seek a second opinion or, because there may be no other choice, reluctantly say "yes."

This attitude is not the best mindset with which to begin treatment.

If, however, the opposite happens and the *perceived value* of the treatment plan outweighs the fee, the patient will not only say "yes" to your recommendations—but will do so with the *gratitude* of which Dr. Pankey spoke.

Under these circumstances, the bill is more likely to be paid cheerfully and promptly, and positive word-of-mouth is more likely to occur.

A common mistake is to assume that *value* and *fee* mean the same thing to patients. They don't. A fee is a fee. Value is the total experience.

REALITY CHECK

"Starbucks is a perfect example," says Bill Dickerson, DDS, Las Vegas, NV. "They provide a product—coffee. Yet people are wiling to pay $4 for a 50-cent cup of coffee. Why? Because of the environment, service, and atmosphere. This company created a new market based on the service. I love to go to Starbucks," he says, "because everyone loves their job, they are all so friendly, and it's cool. I could buy an espresso machine and make my own at home but I would be missing out on the 'experience.' Think about creating an experience in your office."[2]

HARD-LEARNED LESSON

"Quality," says consultant Martin "Bud" Schulman, "is a 'perception' of the patient and is to a great degree unrelated to the actual quality of the dental work that is provided by the practice. Thus it can be described as being subjective in nature. All of the impressions created by the doctor, staff members, the office decor, the promptness of appointments, and even such things as the landscaping around the office building and parking availability go into that perception."[3]

FROM THE SUCCESS FILES

"When treatment is completed," says Greg Tarantola, DDS, Miami, FL, "we do a post treatment consultation to review before, during, and after. Talk about building value and putting yourself at the 'top of consciousness!'"[4]

120 Enhance patients' perception of value

A patient judges the "value" of care received in your office by a variety of factors. Among these factors is the *perceived competency* of you and your staff.

"Dental care is not dental care, and quality of service differs enormously," says Gordon Christensen, DDS, MSD, PhD, Provo, UT. "Practitioners who have prepared to deliver high-quality service through graduate or post-graduate education, or long, successful experience, and who have demonstrated superior quality of care, certainly deserve higher fees than practitioners who provide average service. Also some practitioners use the higher quality materials, devices, and equipment to help produce higher-quality services, while others purposely buy less expensive materials or laboratory work."[5]

HARD-LEARNED LESSON

Charge patients for what you do based on your overhead, time, and expertise—*especially* your expertise.

ACTION STEP

One way to make patients aware of the increasing depth and breadth of your expertise is to include on your Web site, patient newsletter, or reception area bulletin board a listing of the continuing education programs attended by you and your staff.

FROM THE SUCCESS FILES

A patient newsletter from the office of Albert Ousborne, DDS, Thomas Keller, DDS, and Patrick Ousborne, DDS, Towson, MD, contains a schedule of 34 continuing education programs taken in the last year. Courses on local anesthetics, implants, infection control and barrier protection, periodontology, traumatic dental injuries, composite restorations, occlusion, management of the oral cancer patient, and CPR certification are included, among others.[6]

REALITY CHECK

"As long as the patient believes in you, believes you have talent, believes that you have the skill that's needed, and they like you, they will pay your fee," says consultant/speaker James Pride, DDS.[7]

121 Add value to preventive maintenance visits

"The typical hygiene-recall statement," says consultant/speaker Annette Ashley Linder, BS, RDH, "reads, 'Prophy, exam, bitewings.'" Many patients, she adds, think of a recall appointment as "just a cleaning."

ACTION STEP

To add perceived value, Ms. Linder says, give hygiene patients a detailed printout of the services performed, such as medical history update, blood pressure check, oral cancer screening, and oral hygiene homecare instructions for bacterial-plaque control. "Also provide a detailed list of the free products you give your recall patients."

"Enhancing patient perception," says Ms. Linder, "increases compliance levels and reduces cancellations and appointment failure rates."[8]

REALITY CHECK

"It is obvious," says Rick Willeford, MBA, CPA, CFP, "that patients are aware of your fees, but they are not driven by them, as long as *value* is perceived."[9]

122 Hard-learned lessons about discounted fees

Low fees are thought by some dentists to be a significant competitive advantage in attracting new patients. And for the short term, they are. The long-term reality, however, is that regardless of how low your fees are someone will always be willing to do what you do at a lower fee. The winner will be the practice with the deepest pockets and the longest staying power.

A 10%-15% fee differential is almost never the reason that patients change from one practice to another. In many cases, their decisions are based on emotional factors including trust, confidence, rapport, likability, and perceived value.

I've seen more practices hurt by fees that were *too low* than I have by fees that were *too high*.

"Many dentists think having fees lower than those charged by a neighboring dentist," says speaker Dick Barnes, DDS, "will attract more patients. I can tell you it won't affect your patient flow at all unless you're catering to 'shoppers' who want to know the price of everything and the value of nothing. Fees that are too low often cause you to compromise the quality of your dentistry. Don't lock yourself in so tightly with the fees you quote that you're unable to do your very best under all circumstances. Provide quality service and a quality product and there'll always be patients who need your services."[10]

123 Clarify before you contend or compromise

Do patients ever act surprised when quoted a fee? Or react by saying, "That seems very high," or words to that effect? Dentists and staff members whom I've interviewed tell me they respond in a variety of ways to such reactions. Some become defensive. Some offer a reduction for payment in advance. Others offer extended payment options or possibly a less costly alternative treatment. In many cases, these contentions and compromises are premature, if not unnecessary.

ACTION STEP

First, *clarify* what the patient is saying. "That seems very high," for example, could mean any of the following: "It's not worth it. It's more than my neighbor paid for the same thing. It's more than I can afford. It's more than I thought it would be."

Each of these interpretations requires an entirely different response. All that may be needed to clarify the situation is a simple question such as "What makes you say that?" or "Why do you say that?"

REALITY CHECK

"There's a huge difference," says consultant/author Sandy Roth, "between the patient who does not think the service is worth the fee, the patient who does believe it's worth it but has a cash flow problem, and the patient who simply cannot afford the service no matter how many payments you arrange. When you and your staff understand the distinction between these three sets of circumstances," Ms. Roth adds, "you have the opportunity to work with each patient differently. Cash flow may be the problem for many patients, but it isn't the problem for everyone. Some just don't believe that dentistry is important."[11]

124 A disturbing trend

Harris Interactive, a worldwide market research and consulting firm, published a report titled *Haggling With Health Care Providers About Their Prices Likely to Increase Sharply as Out-of-Pocket Costs Rise.*[12]

The report indicates that as healthcare costs have risen, a sizable minority of the public has been talking to healthcare providers to try to negotiate lower bills. For example, 17% have talked to a pharmacist in the last 12 months to pay a lower price, 13% have done the same with physicians, 12% with dentists, and 10% with hospitals. How successful were they? "Approximately half of those who tried to negotiate a lower price, report they did so successfully."

"Our new data," the report adds, "strongly suggest that rising out-of-pocket costs are likely to result in much more consumer negotiation over health care bills and prices over the next few years."

REALITY CHECK

As I wrote at the time of the contest, "It was impossible to single out one perfect response.* Perhaps there is none. Perhaps there is also another factor at work: the emotional bond that dentists have with their patients. The stronger it is, the more they will trust you and accept a simple, straightforward explanation of such matters."[15]

---

127 If you hate discussing fees with patients

You're not alone.

Many (if not most) dentists dislike discussing fees, especially complaints about fees, UCR issues, payment options, and most emphatically, fees that involve "haggling" in any form. Fees that patients readily accept and pay cheerfully and promptly are, of course, another matter.

ACTION STEP

An increasing number of dentists are *delegating* such discussions to treatment or financial coordinators (who are usually women). Among the reasons are the following:

Patients, many of whom are women, are more comfortable discussing fees with another woman or "as one working woman to another" than they are with a doctor (male or female). "They're just more understanding" is the way many patients express it in focus groups.

Staff members are less likely to make concessions, round off fees, or offer discounts to friends of the doctor than is the doctor. Dentists and staff members agree that the totals are invariably higher when treatment or financial coordinators make the financial arrangements.

Collections improve when the person making the initial arrangements also is responsible for collections. There can't be any "He/she said I shouldn't worry about the bill" excuse for not paying in a timely manner.

---

*In lieu of a contest prize, a donation was made to the American Fund for Dental Health.

What's the best way to delegate this task? Simply explain your clinical findings and recommendations to patients and then let your treatment or financial coordinator handle the discussion of the costs involved, the payment options, and any questions the patient may have.

Delegate fee discussions selectively or otherwise, depending on how much you hate discussing fees with patients.

REALITY CHECK

Surprisingly, some staff members also dislike fee discussions, and the accounts receivable in such offices are invariably higher than necessary. This can be avoided by asking job applicants: "How do you feel about asking people for money?"

128　Hard-learned lessons about raising fees

As consultant Bud Ham has said, it doesn't make sense to provide clinical excellence and charge for mediocrity.

By the same token, high fees in a shabby, understaffed office don't work.

The two-word formula to reduce complaints about fees is *no surprises*. Inform before you perform.

If you never get complaints about fees, it means either that you and your staff are providing quality care and first-rate service and your patients think it's worth every penny, *or* you're undercharging.

Resist knocking dentists who have lower fees with the "apples versus oranges" argument. In addition to legal and ethical considerations, it may sound like sour grapes. It's better to acknowledge that your fees are higher. Then explain, if necessary, that the services you and your staff provide require more time and attention to detail than lower fees would allow. The *implication* is that your services are superior.

"The plain fact is," says consultant/speaker Bill Rossi, "that demand for dentistry is not very fee-sensitive. That is, charging less than average won't get you lots of patients and charging more than average won't drive away patients."[16]

"Phobic patients take more time to treat," says Jack Bynes, DMD, Coventry, CT, "especially at the beginning. You have to charge adequately for your time. Many dentists are fixated on charging per procedure rather than for their time. It isn't fair to you or your patients to charge the same amount for a one-surface restoration that takes 20 minutes as opposed to one that takes 40 minutes to accomplish. Establishing more than one fee schedule and assigning patients to a particular schedule based on your estimate of the time needed is necessary."[17]

"If you don't charge what you're worth," says William G. Dickerson, DDS, FAGD, Las Vegas, NV, "you become what you're worth."[18]

People will tolerate higher fees for dentists with excellent reputations.

"Raising fees," says consultant/speaker Charles Blair, DDS, "is one decision that should be thought about less, rather than more. Doctors should not be paralyzed by the fear that raising fees will adversely affect their practice. Based on our experience over the past 25+ years, we have yet to see a single practitioner who increased his or her fees to a desired percentile, or who implemented an across the board increase of 10 percent or less, that actually registered a decline in practice profitability the following year."[19]

When you raise fees, should you give patients advance notice? Write letters with explanations about escalating costs? Post bulletin board notices? The consensus of dentists with whom I've spoken is "Just *do* it."

Remember, if you raise fees, you're no under no obligation to maintain them. If there are signs of significant resistance, you can, and possibly should, reduce fees to their previous levels, but first do the math. Sometimes, less is more.

In all the years I've been surveying dentists on the subject, I've met only a handful who raised their fees and later regretted it. Most regret they hadn't done it *sooner*.

REALITY CHECK

"Take a long, hard look at your fees," says consultant/speaker David Schwab, PhD. "It's no secret that overhead costs in dental offices have been rising steadily. You need to set realistic fees that enable you to pay a top-notch staff excellent wages, have state-of-the-art equipment and a first-rate office, spend quality time with each patient and not feel pressured to overbook yourself, and in the final analysis, generate a reasonable profit."[20]

ACTION STEP

If you've neglected to raise your fees for several years, now might be the time to make a major adjustment. Because you've been under-charging, you may have attracted a number of price-sensitive patients. To counterbalance these patients, go ahead and increase your fees, but tell your current patients that they'll continue to pay the old rate as a reward for their loyalty. At the end of some predetermined period, dis-continue the courtesy discount. Yes, you'll lose some bargain hunters, but you'll replace them with less price-sensitive patients who will help keep your practice healthy.

129 The high fee paradox

Periodic fee increases do cause some "price-conscious" patients to leave a practice, although dentists invariably report the numbers are less than anticipated. Based on seminar surveys I've conducted, however, some 10%-15% of practices actually *get busier* after a fee increase. There doesn't appear to be a simple explanation; rather, a combination of factors is involved.

Newly acquired expertise, equipment, and office improvements *justify* higher fees. (Patients however, need to be aware of such improvements.)

When dentists and hygienists who charge more for their services also *try harder* to provide above-average patient care and personal atten-tion, patients' expectations (based on past performance) are exceeded, leading to greater patient satisfaction.

Patients (like all consumers) tend to relate *quality* to *cost.* "If you pay more, it's probably *worth* more" is the theory. Obviously, this is only a perception but one that is generally true. Like it or not, some dentists' reputations are based solely on their fees.

When these factors combine in the right proportions and under the right circumstances, they produce increased referrals and practice growth, if not in all cases, at least in the 10%-15% of practices surveyed.

Is this a rationale for raising fees? Definitely not. There are numer-ous other factors to consider. The high-fee paradox, however, is a marketplace phenomenon worth noting.

130 Hard-learned lessons about profitability

"Quality cannot exist without profitability," says Tom McDougal, DDS, Richardson, TX. "A dental practice with an overhead of 70 percent that reduces fees by 15 percent must double productivity to remain at the same level of profitability."[21]

"Profitability can be significantly improved," says Michael Gradeless, DDS, Indianapolis, IN, "if you use a less-expensive dental lab or reduce payroll costs. This is where you must examine your own personal vision of how you want to practice. It is written in my mission statement that our staff will be comprised of the highest-quality individuals who will be highly compensated. If your vision specifies high-quality labs and a well-paid staff, your profitability will be very limited if you participate in reduced-fee dental plans."[22]

"It still is amazing how many doctors have bought into the managed-care promise that by cutting fees, they actually can increase practice profitability through higher volume," says Rick Willeford, MBA, CPA, CFP. "Doctors with the highest-overhead percentages require the biggest increase in revenues to maintain profitability for a given fee cut. For example, a doctor with a 40 percent profit margin institutes a 10 percent fee cut. That doctor must increase his revenues 33 percent to maintain levels of profitability!"

"Few if any doctors," Mr. Willeford says, "can make up the additional volume required to maintain practice profitability following a fee cut. You would be better off phasing out of those programs. Then, raise your fees, increase your marketing efforts, expand the scope of services that you offer—and watch your practice profitability increase dramatically while you eliminate the headaches associated with lower quality, managed care participation."[23]

"Even when doctors are aware of the tremendous impact that raising fees can have on their practice profitability," says consultant/speaker Charles Blair, DDS, "many are still reluctant to act. In order to take decisive action, doctors must overcome the fear that raising fees will actually decrease their practice volume and related profitability due to resistance from insurance companies, staff, and patients alike."

For example, says Dr. Blair, "A doctor who implements a 10 percent fee increase, and whose practice has a 35 percent profit margin (practice overhead is 65 percent) must suffer a 22.3 percent drop in patient volume before his or her practice profit actually declines."[24]

"My suggestion," says author Richard Carlson, PhD, "is to charge what you are truly worth. This realistic yet confident pricing strategy keeps you free from resentment and pointed toward your dreams."[25]

Notes

1. Griffin J, Lowenstein MW. *Customer WinBack: How to Recapture Lost Customers and Keep Them Loyal.* San Francisco: Jossey-Bass, 2001.
2. Dickerson B. Creating the Successful Dental Practice. *Dental Economics,* January 2004, 80, 82, 84, 130.
3. Schulman ML. Change Your Practice Successfully! Rome, NY: Canterbury Press, 2000.
4. Interview with Greg Tarantola, DDS, www.spiritofcaring.com, August 28, 2004.
5. Christensen G. Dental Fees: A Candid Discussion. *Journal of the American Dental Association,* November 1993, 87-88.
6. Ousborne A, Keller T. Continuing Education. *Chairside Chatter,* Spring 2003, 3.
7. Martinsons J. Fearful of Raising Your Fees? *Dental Practice Report,* October 2001, 16-18.
8. Linder AA. It's Bill Paying Season! *Dental Economics,* April 2003, 92.
9. Willeford R. 2002 Practice, Salary, and Fee Surveys, *Dental Economics,* December 2002, 28-44.
10. Barnes D. Dealing With the Fear of Fees. *Aesthetic Dentistry* 2(2), 2.
11. Roth S. Money Talks. *Dental Economics,* November 2003.
12. "Haggling" With Health Care Providers About Their Prices Likely to Increase Sharply as Out-of-Pocket Costs Rise. *Harris Interactive Health Care News,* March 6, 2002, 2, 5.
13. Costello D. Medical Care: Can We Talk Price? *Wall Street Journal,* February 8, 2002, W.1.
14. www.21stcenturydental.com/smith/information.html, August 28, 2004.
15. Levoy B. What Readers Say to Patients About UCR. *Dental Economics,* August 1993, 27-32.
16. Rossi B. Cutting Out The PPOs. *Dental Economics,* March 2001, 68-78.
17. Bynes J. Shaping Your Practice. *Dental Economics,* March 2004, 139-141.
18. Dickerson WG. Why Is Esthetic Dentistry Grouped With the Outlaws? *Dental Economics,* December 1998, 42-46, 105.
19. Doctors Surveyed on Raising Fees. *Blair/McGill Advisory,* December 2000, 3.
20. Schwab D. How to Take Your Practice to the Next Level. *The Personal Report,* 1st Quarter 1999, 2-3.
21. McDougal T. Managing to Care—Not Managed Care. *Dental Economics,* May 1996, 22-24.
22. Gradeless M. We Are Not Wal-Mart. *Dental Economics,* November 2003, 110.
23. Willeford R. 2003 Dental Economics Practice Survey. *Dental Economics,* December 2003, 28-39.
24. Will Raising Fees Hurt Your Practice? *Blair/McGill Advisory,* December 1998.
25. Carlson R. *Don't Worry, Make Money.* New York: Hyperion Press, 1998.

10

Measure What Matters to Patients

"Measure what matters to customers," says Patricia B. Sebold, author of *The Customer Revolution.* "Most companies measure and monitor the significant factors affecting their businesses. But none of these metrics matter to your customers or help you improve your customer's experience in doing business with you. The companies that will be pulling ahead of the pack over the next few years are those that take the quality of their customers' experience very seriously."[1]

The purpose of this chapter about marketing research is to help you learn what you and your staff are doing *right* in your practice as far as patients are concerned, what (if anything) you're doing *wrong*, and what *changes* (if any) need to be made.

131 What's #1?

"We spend in the neighborhood of $10 million a year on market research," says J. Willard (Bill) Marriott, Jr., CEO of the Marriott Corporation. "We believe it is absolutely essential to know the markets we serve and what our guests want from us."[2]

As an example, Marriott Hotels asked 27,000 frequent travelers (their target population) which hotel services they ranked most important. The hotel service most frequently ranked number one was "express check in."

"A 1997 J.D. Power and Associates Airline Customer Satisfaction Study showed that on-time performance was 22 percent of what determined customer satisfaction. No other single element was judged higher than 15 percent."[3]

Without knowing such priorities, management can only guess how to best train their employees to achieve customer satisfaction.

Which aspects of your practice do your best patients rank most important? How should you train your staff to achieve patient satisfaction, referrals, and practice growth?

This chapter will explain numerous ways to obtain such information.

132 Ask a simple question

An outpatient survey from the Williamsport Hospital in Williamsport, PA, asks "Have you used the Williamsport Hospital Services before? If yes, has the quality of the services improved, remained the same, or declined?"

The first principle in the quest for quality is recognition that quality is what the *patient* perceives it to be, not what you or I say it is (or what it *should* be).

REALITY CHECK
How would your returning patients answer such a survey?

133 Monitor patient satisfaction

Monitoring patient satisfaction is essential to the success of high-performance practices, especially if they participate in managed care.

Healthcare organizations are operating in an extremely competitive environment, and patient satisfaction has become critical in gaining and maintaining market share. In addition, these organizations are increasing their reliance on patient satisfaction data to decide which providers to recruit and whether to renew contracts with existing providers. In some cases, bonus payments to providers are linked to patient satisfaction. The reasons are practical. Satisfied members are more likely to re-enroll in a plan, pay more to remain in it, ask their employers to retain a plan, and encourage others to join their plan.

REALITY CHECK

The fact that patients don't complain doesn't necessarily mean they're satisfied with the care they're receiving, the staff members with whom they interact, and the office in general. Current research shows that only 4% of dissatisfied patients even bother to complain, at least to the person who either caused or could remedy the problem. Some are too inhibited to do so, others consider it futile, and some are afraid of being labeled "complainers."

They do, however, complain to others, 10 to 12 on average. In many cases, the patient complains to the person who referred them.

ACTION STEP

A short patient survey provides the "feedback" every practice needs to properly assess patient satisfaction. A few sentences can explain its purpose. The following is an example:

"Dear Patient,

We are interested to know how you and the other patients we serve view our practice and what changes if any you would recommend. We'd be grateful if you would take a few minutes to complete this survey. Your anonymous answers will be most valuable to our ongoing effort to provide friendly, convenient, high-quality care."

The following are some of the questions typically used in these surveys. The first set of questions is from a "long form" and is usually given to patients at the conclusion of their office visits along with a postage-paid envelope. The second set of questions is from a "short form" that patients can more readily complete in the office before leaving.

In addition to the examples on the following page, numerous other questions can be used to monitor patient satisfaction. These are included in the various marketing research techniques discussed on the pages that follow. Choose those that are most appropriate.

To get a representative sampling of patient feedback, I'd recommend having a front desk person periodically distribute 150 to 200 surveys to randomly selected patients over the course of several weeks.

Patient Survey (Long Form)

	Yes	No
Were you scheduled for an appointment within a reasonable amount of time?	____	____
Were you greeted properly when you arrived?	____	____
Were our billing and insurance policies made clear to you?	____	____
Did the doctor listen carefully to your concerns?	____	____
Was the hygienist gentle?	____	____
Did the doctor thoroughly explain his or her findings and recommendations?	____	____
Was the office clean and well kept?	____	____
If a friend were looking for a dentist would you feel comfortable in recommending our practice?	____	____

If you answered "no" to any of the preceding questions,
please briefly explain the reasons _____

_____

_____

Name (optional)

Patient Survey (Short Form)

On a scale of 1 to 5, with 5 signifying the highest degree of importance and satisfaction and 1 the lowest, how would you rate the following aspects of our practice?

How Important Is This To You		How Good Are We At This
1 2 3 4 5	The office environment	1 2 3 4 5
1 2 3 4 5	Our billing and insurance policies	1 2 3 4 5
1 2 3 4 5	Our office hours	1 2 3 4 5
1 2 3 4 5	Our scheduling and punctuality with appointments	1 2 3 4 5
1 2 3 4 5	The attention and care you received from our doctor(s)	1 2 3 4 5

Name (optional)_____

You'll most likely get more short forms returned than long ones, but if written answers are included, the latter will yield more information. Consider distributing some of each or perhaps alternating them for follow-up surveys.

Another alternative is to include a patient survey on your practice Web site.

TWO MAJOR BENEFITS

You'll obtain valuable feedback about how your practice is perceived and perhaps some surprises that you're doing far better (or worse) than you realized. You may also learn (from the short form) that certain aspects of your practice are more (or less) important to patients than you thought. Regardless of the outcome, these patient surveys will alert your staff to the importance you place on patient satisfaction and their role in achieving it.

Patient satisfaction data are receiving increasing attention from managed care organizations, consumers, employers, and accrediting organizations. Don't risk being the last to know what your patients are thinking and saying.

FROM THE SUCCESS FILES

Based on the results of 10,000 patient satisfaction surveys conducted during a 2-year period, Akron General Medical Center in Akron, OH, determined that the highest correlation to quality as defined by patients is its staff's ability to be sensitive to patient needs. On making this determination, Akron General decided to provide customer service training to its nurses and other employees with direct patient contact, as well as to managers.[4]

134 A one-question survey

"Could customer satisfaction surveys be reduced to a single question?" asks consultant/author Frederick F. Reichheld in the *Harvard Business Review.* "If so, what would that question be?"

"It took two years of research to figure that out," Reichheld says, "research that linked survey responses with actual customer behavior—purchasing patterns and referrals—and ultimately with company growth. The results were clear yet counterintuitive. It turned out that a single survey question can in fact serve as a useful predictor of growth. But that question isn't about customer satisfaction or even loyalty, at least in so many words. Rather, it's about customers' willingness to recommend a product or service to someone else. In fact, in most of the industries that I studied, the percentage of customers who were enthusiastic enough to refer a friend or colleague—perhaps the strongest sign of customer loyalty—correlated directly with differences in growth rates among competitors."[5]

The single question that emerged from Reichheld's research was "How likely is it that you would recommend (Company X) to a friend or colleague?" using a scale of 0 to 10 to measure responses (10, extremely likely to recommend; 5, neutral; and 0, not at all likely). Those customers that gave ratings of 9 or 10 were labeled "promoters." Reichheld concluded that creating more of these promoters would be a sure path to increased growth and greater profitability.

ACTION STEP

Although I don't recommend replacing patient satisfaction surveys with a single question, I do strongly advocate *reducing* the number of questions found in extremely lengthy practice surveys that examine every little detail of a patient's visit and that, in many cases, wear people out before they can complete them.

Significant data from Reichheld's research suggest, however, that this one question should at least be on patient surveys, and perhaps should be the first question.

As far as cultivating more of what Reichheld calls "promoters," see Chapter 7.

135 Focus groups

Long used in qualitative market research about consumer products, focus groups are beginning to be used by dentists to view their practices through the eyes of patients.

A typical focus group consists of eight to ten invited patients who meet for 1 to 1 1/2 hours, usually in the evening, to talk specifically about the practice. The ideal participants are astute, verbal, and willing to speak up about the practice. The preferred setting is a small conference room in a hotel or private room in a restaurant. Light refreshments such as coffee and cake or fruit and cheese are typically served.

Many patients will be pleased to participate without compensation Others will be more interested if an incentive is offered, such as a credit against future services.

TESTED TIPS

The ideal person to conduct the session is a professional focus group facilitator who, by definition, is neutral about the practice and more likely to make the participants comfortable enough to express their true feelings, for better or for worse. To locate such a facilitator, contact a school of business at a local college. A professor or perhaps a graduate student may be available, or you can look in the Yellow Pages under "marketing" or "marketing research."

The facilitator should have strong interpersonal skills and be able to start the discussion and then listen without interrupting or getting defensive. He or she should also be strong enough to manage the direction of the discussion while making sure that low-key individuals are not overwhelmed by more outspoken participants.

The following types of questions can be used to start the discussion:

"In your experience with the practice, what have you liked?" (It's best to start with a question that everyone will find easy to answer.)

"What if anything have you disliked?" (Patients may at first be hesitant to answer. Be patient. Someone will speak up and then others will follow.)

"Why did you choose this practice above all others?"

"Can you think of specific situations that you wish the staff had handled differently?"

"Have there been situations that you wish the doctor had handled differently?"

"How do you feel about the office environment? Could it be improved in any way?"

"How about the office hours? Appointment scheduling?"

Action Step

Do you want more children in your practice? Older patients? 35-50 year-old career people? Women? Candidates for cosmetic dentistry? Other target populations? Consider focus groups consisting of patients from each of these constituencies. Each will have its own point of view, likes, and dislikes.

Suggestion

You'll get better results if the group is homogenous in terms of education and socioeconomic status. People will be more at ease with each other, more willing to participate in the discussion.

Reality Check

Charles R. Atwood, MD, a pediatrician in Crowley, LA, says about focus groups, "No matter how much you invite honesty, some people just won't tell you things they're afraid you don't want to hear. So at the end of each focus group, I pass out index cards and ask patients to write any comments, opinions, or criticisms they haven't already expressed—things they'd rather suggest anonymously. Over the years, I've received some doozies."[6]

---

136 Advisory board

To help in long-range planning, many practitioners create Advisory Boards consisting of patients that Albert Ousborne, Jr., DDS, Towson, MD, recommends should "have the traits, attitudes, and values that you would like to see more of in your practice."

Here's how he does it. Dr. Ousborne arranges for a 3-hour session in a private room at a local restaurant or country club to which 15 "ideal patients" are invited for brunch (on a Saturday) or dinner on a weekday evening.

After the meal, Dr. Ousborne holds a 2-hour meeting at which the participants are given a series of questions and invited to provide "brutally" honest answers. The tables are arranged in a horseshoe or full-square shape so everyone has direct visual contact.

Suggested questions include the following:

When asking such a question, it's important to hold eye contact with the patient and look genuinely interested. Otherwise the patient may not attach any importance to the question and simply say "fine."

Regardless of what you hear—brickbats or bouquets—the feedback you obtain from such interviews will help you identify hidden "blind spots" about your practice.

139 Mystery shoppers

In the context of professional practice, "mystery shoppers" are really *mystery patients*, anonymous evaluators who provide insights into how well everyone in the practice, from receptionist to doctor, is serving patients.

Here's how an ophthalmology practice did it.

Suzanne Bruno, ophthalmic administrator of Horizon Eye Care, Margate, NJ, recruited mystery patients to visit their five offices and surgery center. All were members of a local civic association, but only she knew who they were. The practice made a charitable donation to the civic group and provided complimentary exams and 50% discounts on eyewear to all participants.

A few of the mystery shoppers, including two who needed cataract surgery, were already patients in the practice. The rest were new patients, most of whom stayed with the practice. They paid for their visits and were reimbursed on the receipts. It took a huge effort on Ms. Bruno's part to develop the lengthy questionnaire she distributed to the mystery shoppers, communicate secretly with these patients, process all their refunds, and compile evaluations. But the feedback has been invaluable.

For example, being "child friendly" was a practice goal, so some of the volunteers were asked to bring their children in for exams. "We discovered," Ms. Bruno says, "that our staff and our doctors were good with children but our office wasn't. That's one thing we changed as a direct result of the program. All our offices now have toy boxes with books, toys, and even video games for older children."[8]

ACTION STEP

The following are a few of the questions you can provide mystery shoppers to evaluate your practice:

"Was the phone answered within three rings?"

"How long did you have to wait for an appointment?"

"Were you greeted promptly when you entered the office?"

"How long did you wait before being seen by the dentist or hygienist?"

"Did you feel uncomfortable with any person on the staff?"

"Was the facility spotlessly clean?"

"Were you given an opportunity to ask the dentist or hygienist questions?"

"Were new procedures explained clearly?"

"How would you rate the professionalism of the dentist and staff?"

140 Critique yourself

Question: After a treatment conference, what percent of your recommendations are *accepted* by patients? If it's not as high as you'd like, one reason may have to do with *how* you say *what* you say to patients.

REALITY CHECK

You probably haven't had your communication skills critiqued in a long time, if ever. The truth is, no one is likely to tell you about your shortcomings as a communicator. The easiest, most practical way to learn how you come across to others is to audit yourself by *tape recording* your interactions with patients. You may be highly pleased with what you hear, *or* you may be taken aback.

Either way, it's worth a listen.

Among the *communication blunders* you may unintentionally be making are the following:

• *Using overly technical language.* Doctors often explain their findings and recommendations in language that patients don't understand. Rather than admit it and look foolish, many patients just nod their heads and pretend to understand.

REALITY CHECK

Gregory Kaveney, Executive Director of the Seattle-King County (Washington) Dental Society, tells me his office averages 3 to 4 calls a day from patients who don't understand the procedures their dentists have recommended.

What's troubling isn't just the number of calls. It's the number of patients who are confused, *not calling*, and not following through on needed treatment.

- *Being too rushed.* When explaining the importance of replacing a missing posterior tooth for the five hundredth time (especially if you're time pressured) it's easy to fall into the trap of speaking-so-fast-that-patients-can't-follow. Again, some patients will pretend to understand when in fact, they don't.

Patients can't accept what they don't understand.

- *Talking too much.* Another well-intentioned habit that no one is ever going to tell you about is the tendency to talk too much, telling patients *more* than they want to know or *need to know* about the etiology of chronic, inflammatory periodontal disease.

Listen to yourself. You may start to squirm as you hear yourself going on and on and on and on and on.

- *Using high-pressure tactics.* It's natural to want patients to accept your recommendations. But continuing to "sell" after patients say "no" or "I'd like to think about it" may come across as "pushy." What you say may be well intentioned, but if it is *perceived* as "high-pressure," it will undermine trust and make patients uncomfortable.

The issue is not how technical, rushed, talkative, or high-pressure you *are*, but rather how technical, rushed, talkative, or high-pressure you're *perceived* to be.

ACTION STEP

Audit yourself to learn if you're as good a communicator as you think you are.

HARD-LEARNED LESSON

In order to learn from mistakes, you first have to recognize you are making mistakes.

Caveat. The permissibility of taping a conversation without a patient's knowledge and consent varies from state to state. Check with your attorney to learn what obligations if any, you have in this regard

141 Questions for specialists to pursue with family dentists

Specialists need to measure not only what matters to patients but also what matters to their referring dentists.

The following is a composite of written surveys used by periodontists that can be adapted for any of the dental specialties.

Questionnaire for Referring Dentists

Name _____

Has my treatment of your patients met your expectations?

Would you like a copy of my diagnosis and treatment plan? Would you prefer a brief clinical report or a longer narrative?

What is the best time to reach you by telephone?

How often would you like progress evaluations during a patient's active periodontal treatment? (bimonthly, monthly, after each visit?)

Would you be interested in having me or a staff member present a program on any topic related to periodontics? (List suggested topics.) Would you prefer a staff meeting or a seminar/workshop?

Would a brochure that explains periodontal treatment be helpful for patients who are scheduled for periodontal treatment and/or those you would like to motivate to start treatment?

Would you prefer that referrals to other specialists be made by me or by you?

What are your thoughts about maintenance visits to increase a patient's chance of periodontal stability? (a) all with you? (b) all with me? (c) alternate? (d) at our discretion?

Would a newsletter about recent advancements in periodontics be of interest?

Can you identify any problems you, your staff, or patients might have had with our practice?

REALITY CHECK

Don't be surprised if referring dentists have widely different needs, interests, and priorities. The more that you and your staff can accommodate their individual preferences, the better your relationships will be.

HARD-LEARNED LESSON

"Simply creating a brand is not good enough for today's sophisticated consumers," say Renée M. Zakoor and Hal E. Quinley, partner and executive vice president, respectively, of Yankelovich Partners Inc., Claremont, CA. "The brand has to be constantly monitored to ensure that it is delivering its intended promise. Brand maintenance is critical to building a strong brand image; a strong image is the ultimate competitive weapon against the muddle and overload that exist in the consumer marketplace. A strong, trustworthy brand helps forge closer relationships with consumers, enhances brand equity, and opens the door for greater business opportunities."[9]

Notes

1. Sebold PB. *The Customer Revolution.* New York, Crown Publishing, 2000.
2. Back to School. *Incentive,* March 1993, 25.
3. Krauss P. *The Book of Management Wisdom: Classic Writings by Legendary Managers.* New York: John Wiley & Sons, Inc., 2000.
4. Development Dimensions International, http://www.ddiworld.com/real_solutions/akrongeneral.asp, August 28, 2004.
5. Reichheld FF. The One Number You Need to Grow. *Harvard Business Review,* December 2003, 46-54.
6. Atwood, CR. Give These Little Extras and Watch Your Practice Grow. *Medical Economics,* March 1992, 133-143.
7. Ousborne AL, Jr. Create Your LAB and Then Listen! *Dental Economics,* August 2003, 34.
8. Beiting J. Taking the Mystery Out of Patient Satisfaction. *Quirk's Marketing Research Review,* January 2001, 16, 48-49.
9. www.yankelovich.com, August 28, 2004.

11

Get the Right People
on Board

The hiring of employees is the single most important management task you do. In fact, says Phillip Bonner, DDS, FACD, Editor-In-Chief of *Dentistry Today,* "The importance of the dental office staff cannot be overemphasized. A staff that is knowledgeable, efficient, and enthusiastic about their jobs can literally make the difference between a failing practice and one that is successful in all aspects, from quality of patient care to financial health."[1]

The first step: Get the right people on board.

142 Hire people who fit the culture of your practice

Knowledge and skills are, of course, important traits when hiring new employees. Equally important are people who will be a good fit with the *culture* of your practice.

Culture refers to the core values and shared beliefs that develop within a practice and guide the behavior of its team members.

In their book *Corporate Cultures: The Rites and Rituals of Corporate Life,* Terrence E. Deal and Alan A. Kennedy write, "If employees know what their company stands for, if they know what standards they are to uphold, then they are much more likely to make decisions that will support those standards. They are also more likely to feel as if they are an important part of the organization. They are motivated because the company has meaning for them."[2]

"Hire compatible people," says John A. Wilde, DDS, Keokuk, IA. "The key point in the entire employment process is to hire people whose values mirror yours and those of the practice, and whom you like."[3]

When there's a good fit between the culture of a practice and its employees, people tend to be happier, harder working, more productive, and, as a rule, they stick around longer.

Bernard Marcus, one of the co-founders of Home Depot, was interviewed about his company's corporate culture for the book *Management*. "It starts with the basics," he says, "hiring the right people, the folks in the store who will create the shopping environment. We want extroverts, people who like other people. We look for people with pleasing personalities and people who are highly motivated and want to learn. You have to be discerning to find them. Typically, out of 8,000 applicants, we hire 200 people."[4]

Herb Kelleher, CEO of Southwest Airlines, was similarly asked about his company's corporate culture. "It starts with the hiring," he said. "We are zealous about hiring. We look for a particular type of person, regardless of which category it is. We look for attitudes that are positive and for people who can lend themselves to causes. We want folks who have a good sense of humor and people who are interested in performing as a team and take joy in team results instead of individual accomplishments."[5]

In both of these examples, the top management of the companies was highly focused on the type of person best suited to the long-term goals of their organizations.

FROM THE SUCCESS FILES

Gulf Breeze Hospital is an acute-care facility in Gulf Breeze, FL, that ranked in 2001 among the top 2% in patient satisfaction surveys. Its 280 staff members are trained to make three major pledges to ensure outstanding service to patients. "It all begins," says the hospital's administrator, Dick Fulford, "with a positive attitude."

Never say, "It's not my job."

Reduce and eliminate hassles.

Provide personalized professional care.

"Fulford says that every person working at the hospital has the opportunity to make a patient's interaction exceptional. Applicants are immediately told that if they can't make this commitment, they will probably not fit in with the Gulf Breeze Hospital culture."[6]

143 Begin the search

To begin the search for employees who are compatible with the culture of your practice, first get a solid handle on the core values of your practice as discussed in Chapter 3. Then when interviewing job applicants, ask questions and make observations that enable you to learn about their values, temperament, and job-related priorities.

"After the interview," says Kenneth R. James, DDS, Kent, WA, "ask yourself whether the interviewee warrants a positive answer to these three questions:"

"Does he or she fit into our office culture?"

"Does his or her temperament suit those of the other people in our office?"

"Does he or she fit comfortably in our office environment?"[7]

If you make a mistake and hire team members who don't fit the culture of your practice, it will become readily apparent to everyone concerned, in which case, it's best to just cut your losses and move on.

REALITY CHECK

Most dental practices have unique cultures in the same way that employees have job-related priorities. And these preferences are neither good nor bad. They're just different. Those differences are part of what makes some practices (and some employees) more or less attractive to one another.

Beyond skills and experience, what are some of the traits that leading practitioners look for in a new employee?

144 Qualities of exceptional employees

The following are some of the qualities that Steven L. Rasner, DMD, Cherry Hill, NJ, finds in exceptional employees:

"Perceives himself or herself as a 'winner.' Look for clues that speak of one's pursuit of individual excellence."

"Eagerness to learn. Not all candidates have lifestyles or a desire that will embrace continued education. Make it clear that your office seeks candidates who embrace the magic of learning."

"Needs to work. Staff members who need to work historically have been more interested in the team values we profess and the commitment needed in and out of the office to attain high levels of achievement."

"An infectious smile. People who are internally happy often carry a glow that reveals itself in a relaxed, natural, and almost infectious smile. Someone once said that the morale of your office will only be as good as your worst attitude. Keep the winners—pass up the frowns."[8]

145 Hire "people" employees

"Hire 'people' employees," says William G. Dickerson, DDS, FAACD, Las Vegas, NV. "Technical skills are less important than good personalities and attitudes. Skills can be taught, whereas personalities are usually unchangeable. 'High-on-life' attitudes and team players are the grease to keep the wheels turning smoothly and effectively. A highly-skilled, know-it-all matriarch or pessimistic introvert is more destructive to your practice than an optimistic and enthusiastic trainee."[9]

FROM THE SUCCESS FILES
Ann Rhoades, Southwest Airlines former vice president of people (her actual job title), says, "We tended to hire people with empathy. We wanted to treat passengers as individuals, not numbers on a boarding pass. When we hired people, we asked them to give us an example from their previous job of how they treated a customer who had a problem, and how they made it a win-win situation. We hired only those people who could give us examples of how they treated customers the way we like ours to be treated."[10]

146 Loyalty is #1

Charles Blair, DDS, a management consultant in Charlotte, NC, searches for employees with the following traits, beginning with what he considers the most important:

Loyalty
Stability
Enthusiasm
Judgment
Intelligence
Technical ability

Surprised that the top-ranked characteristics are so subjective? "Creating a conscientious, effective, and efficient team," says Dr. Blair, "depends more on those personality traits than on IQ, computer literacy, or credentials."[11]

147 A sparkling personality who lights up the room

"Hire one person based on entertainment value alone," says author/consultant Nate Booth, DDS, Oceanside, CA. "Find that special person who has a sparkling personality that lights up the room when he or she walks in. In my practice, that person was Susie, a 4 foot, 10 inch bundle of charm. She was our office 'floater.' One of her duties was to escort patients back to the treatment rooms. She was notorious for putting her arms around teenage boys and saying, 'Gee, you're getting so big and strong. You must drive all the girls crazy.' When she was out of the office for a day, everybody would ask, 'Where's Susie?'"[12]

148 Psychological hardiness

Most service-quality gurus say that hiring is the first and most critical step in building a customer-friendly company. "You need to be selective," says Ron Zemke, president of Performance Research Associates in Minneapolis, MN. "It's a lot easier to start with people who've got the right personality qualities to work with customers than it is to struggle to teach those skills to whoever walks in the door."

Zemke says the key indicator of customer-service potential is "a high level of what mental-health professionals call 'psychological hardiness'—qualities such as optimism, flexibility, and the ability to handle stressful situations or criticism without feeling emotionally threatened. Those, of course, are good qualities in many jobs. But experts note that the personality of a customer-service maven may be markedly different from those of achievers in other business venues. Verbal eloquence and persuasiveness, for example, aren't as important as the ability to listen."[13]

149 Involve your staff in the hiring process

Allow your staff to interview job applicants and narrow the list down to a few from which you will make the final selection. Or let your staff have the final approval of someone you've tentatively decided to hire.

If the staff shares in the selection of a new employee, their commitment to the new employee will be stronger. They'll be pulling for the newcomer to succeed because they shared in the hiring decision. Moreover, the team's acceptance of the new staff member helps the newcomer to quickly acquire skills necessary to function effectively as part of the team.

"Set aside time for the candidate to interact with your staff, and even work with them on an office procedure," says Stephen J. Persichetti, DDS, FAGD, an associate professor of practice management at the Oregon Health & Science University School of Dentistry. "This will let you get a better feel for their personality and how well they mesh with your current employees."[14]

Consultant James R. Pride, DDS, Novato, CA, recommends that the staff have a 20-minute meeting or 1-hour lunch (paid for by you) with each of the two or three top candidates. "The purpose of this interview," he says. "is to glean information the applicant might not reveal to you. The staff prepares work-related questions to discover the applicant's motivation and concerns, such as: 'What do you think of the interview process so far?' 'What things might be a concern for you?' and 'What can I tell you about our practice?' The staff's input is important," says Dr. Pride, "however, the final decision remains yours."[15]

150 Don't skimp on payroll

The job of receptionist in a dental office is anything but an entry-level job, as some dentists unfortunately view it. This person is the first contact patients have with your practice. This is also the person with whom referring dentists, physicians, pharmacists and other professional colleagues talk when calling your office.

A Midwestern oral surgeon, realizing how apprehensive many of his patients are when first calling his office, decided such calls (as well as those from referring dentists) must be handled with the utmost diplomacy and skill. And, he concluded, the people most likely to have the training, experience, and personality traits needed for the job were airline flight attendants. They have the know-how to deal with emergencies of all kinds. They also have great people skills, are hard-working, are quick to learn, and are used to on-the-job teamwork.

He found the perfect candidate who, after years of international travel, was ready to settle down. Compared with the standard pay for a dental receptionist, her salary is significantly higher. "But," he said, "it's the best investment I've ever made in my practice."

HARD-LEARNED LESSON

"Hire the best," says management consultant Charles Blair, DDS, Charlotte, NC. "Top practices always recruit the highest quality employees, even though they cost a little more. Despite the higher cost, they represent an excellent value since their productivity far exceeds that received from cheaper, but more mediocre employees."[16]

151 Creatively recruit new employees

Finding the right people for your practice who have positive attitudes, exceptional people skills, and are able to leap tall buildings in a single bound isn't easy. If the usual recruiting channels aren't producing qualified candidates, consider the following alternatives:

"Go to your successful hires," says author Carolyn B. Thompson, "and ask them 'What initially attracted you to us?' and 'What are the factors that make you want to stay with us?' 'Where did you hear about us?' You'll find that a significant number of your employees heard about you from the same sources, such as current or former employees, their friends, or the local newspaper. This is immediate feedback. It will help you to stop wasting money on advertising in the wrong areas You'll find out what is important to the staff: salaries, working relationships, working environment or flexibility for example."[17]

If the salary plus benefits you're offering is lower than the going rate in your area, that might explain the small pool of applicants. A higher salary may produce more and better-qualified applicants. Nothing is more important to patient satisfaction and practice growth than having the right people on board. In the long run, the investment will pay off.

Consider offering a recruiting bonus of $300 to $500 to any staff member who recommends an individual who is subsequently hired after a 90-day probationary period. If an employee you respect likes someone well enough to recommend him or her, the odds are better than average that the new person will fit in with your staff.

At the outset, make it clear that the same high standards and selection process will be used to evaluate job applicants recommended by staff members. Stating this policy up front helps avoid any obligation you may feel to hire someone you don't consider the best choice for your practice

"Run an unusual and eye-catching ad," says Victoria Farr, DDS, Vacaville, CA. "We want the reader to be curious and to know that our office is different." One of their ads reads:

"Our progressive, unique dental team is waiting for a friendly, experienced, fun-loving RDA looking for a new frontier. Please fax your resume . . ."[18]

If one of your *patients* has all the traits you're looking for in an employee, consider recruiting him or her. You might ask, "I'd love to have someone with your personality working here. Do you know of anyone?" The person may be interested in the job or know someone who might be. I know of many dental staff members who were hired in exactly this way.

If you've tried these strategies without success, it may be time to take a second look at the reputation your practice has as a place to work. What, for example, do your employees say about your practice when they gather with their friends at weekend barbecues and describe what it's like to work there? Are they saying what you want them to say? Do you come off as an "Employer of Choice?" If not, then you'll need to ascertain the underlying problems and resolve them (see Chapter 12).

FROM THE SUCCESS FILES

"It has been our experience that our Web site is wonderful for attracting new, high-quality staff members," says orthodontist Kambiz Moin, DMD, MPH, Manchester, NH. "In our newspaper ads, we encourage applicants to visit our Web site in order to learn more about our office and help them make a more informed career decision."[19]

152 Use part-time employees

If you answer "yes" to one or more of the following questions, your practice may benefit from hiring *part-time employees*:

- Have you had difficulty finding qualified, full-time office personnel?
- Does your practice have peaks and valleys of activity?
- Does your staff lack the time to implement ideas that would generate practice growth?
- Do your employees have child or elder care obligations that impinge on their work schedule?

- Has burnout become a problem for any of your employees?
- Has employee turnover been a problem in your practice?

In many areas of the country, part-time employees are the fastest growing segment of the labor force. Among the many benefits of hiring them are the following:

- An increase in the pool of applicants including those who may have left the profession to start a family, and now want to return to work on a part-time basis.
- A tremendous recruitment edge when other practices offer the same compensation but no part-time option.
- A leveling of the peaks and valleys of workflow and improvement in patient service at the busiest times.
- Improved productivity and morale. Because of a reduced workweek, part-time employees bring increased energy to the job. They're also able to better focus on their work and usually miss fewer days.
- Retention of older employees who have valuable skills and experience. Surveys indicate many members of this age group would extend their working life *if* they could work part-time, rather than choose between full-time work and retirement.
- Reduction of labor costs during slow times when full-time employees are not needed. Also, as a general rule, employers are not required under current law to provide fringe benefits for employees who work fewer than 1000 hours a year. Check your state's requirements.

One Caveat. Part-time employees may feel like outsiders or "second class" citizens. To foster a connection, schedule staff meetings at times so they can attend, keep them informed about policy and protocol changes, and provide frequent performance feedback.

153 Offer family-friendly perks

FACTS
50 percent of all mothers with children less than one year old are in the work force. 25 percent of the work force have elder care responsibilities. In both cases, the numbers are increasing.

Studies show that staff members with such caretaking responsibilities tend to come to work late, use the telephone excessively for personal calls, have more absenteeism, and quit their jobs more readily. The buzzword to accommodate such employees in what *Business Week* calls the "new world of work" is *flexibility*.

After a recent seminar, a dental assistant told me, "When my father died two years ago, my boss said, 'Don't worry about your work. Don't think about the office. Think only about yourself and your family. If you need a week or even two weeks, take it. We'll cover for you.'"

"It wasn't the first time that the chips were down," she added, "and he was there for me, putting my needs first. It meant a lot at the time—especially because I understood the pressure he was under as well."

If you're experiencing a shortage of skilled job applicants and/or high employee turnover, consider adding to your package of basic benefits some of the following family-friendly perks now being offered by an increasing number of employers:

- Flextime (flexible work hours)
- Compressed work week (work longer days in exchange for a shorter week)
- Job sharing (divide one full-time job, for example, into two part-time jobs)
- Telecommuting opportunities (work at home with computer, fax, and modem)
- Paid "personal days" to be used for any purpose
- Paid maternity/paternity leave
- On-site child care (e.g., provided by a senior citizen)
- Tuition-paid continuing education
- On-site fitness equipment (e.g., treadmill)
- Staff lounge (with microwave, refrigerator)
- Special areas (other than bathrooms) where working moms can breast-feed their babies. Studies cite a decreased rate of absenteeism where this is allowed.

Family-friendly perks like those mentioned in the preceding list are more effective at retaining valuable employees than cash incentives, according to 352 human resource executives surveyed by the American Management Association.

REALITY CHECK

"It would nice to offer your employees a world of benefits," says Pamela Miller, OD, JD, Highland, CA. "Unfortunately, that's not realistic. So find out what they need most."[20]

ACTION STEP

Conduct one-on-one interviews with employees to learn which of the "perks" that you're willing to offer are of greatest interest.

Family-friendly perks can ease the conflicts many employees have between home and work, reduce turnover, and enhance on-the-job performance. They can also be highly appealing to prospective employees in a tight labor market. These perks should be included in classified ads.

154 Avoid costly hiring mistakes

Have you ever hired someone who sounded great in the interview, and then fell short on the job? What went wrong?

Job seekers have become increasingly savvy and better prepared for job interviews than ever before. There are countless books and Web sites to help them look good on a job interview and get the job they want. In addition, because of the litigious times in which we live, even reference checks may fail to give you the whole story about a job applicant.

I've asked countless personnel managers in a wide range of businesses and professions what interview questions they've found most helpful in judging job applicants. The following is a sampling of such questions. What's good about these questions is that job applicants have no way of knowing the needs of your practice or exactly what *you're* looking for. Their best choice is to be honest and straightforward.

- "What are you looking for in your next job that's missing from your present one?"
- "Do you prefer to work alone or with others? Explain why."
- "What about your work do you find most challenging?"

- "What aspects of your last job did you like best? Least?"
- "What job-related situations have you found most stressful?"
- "What have you found most effective in dealing with such stress?"
- "What do you consider your greatest strengths? Don't be modest."
- "In which of your jobs did you learn the most?"
- "Tell me about the best boss you ever had. What about the worst?"
- "Have you ever seen a dental hygienist or dental assistant/receptionist (depending on the position for which you're hiring) show especially poor judgment? If so, tell me about it."

TESTED TIP

For best results, probe for further information with such follow-up requests as "please explain" or "that's interesting, tell me more."

---

155 Uncover a job applicant's "inner traits"

After considering job skills and experience, many dentists tend to appraise job applicants according to appearance, communication skills, sociability, or personality. Although these are important traits for a dental office, they're not enough.

Far more important than personality and the like are a person's *inner traits*: intelligence, inner drive, attitude toward work, and the ability to get along with others, to name a few. These factors determine whether a person with the right job skills and experience will be right for your practice

The following are more tested interview questions to help elicit information about these inner traits:

"In your last job, what did you do that you're most proud of?"

"In your last job, when you finished your work ahead of schedule, what did you usually do?"

"Do you like someone who gives you a lot of responsibility or someone who provides a lot of supervision?"

"Have you learned any new skills or explored some new field of interest, even a hobby, since leaving school?"

As a final question, consider asking a job applicant, "Is there anything you'd like to discuss that we haven't talked about?" See if the person asks about job content, your expectations, why the last person left, or other related questions that may provide clues to the person's "inner traits."

Long pauses or "no" answers to such questions can be highly revealing.

156 How important is continuing education?

Continuing education (CE) is part of the culture of many dental practices I've visited. Unfortunately, this requirement comes as a surprise to many newly hired staff members who aren't prepared to give CE their time and effort, especially if it involves overnight travel.

ACTION STEP

"Ideally, you should detail CE and associated travel expectations as part of the *hiring* process," says *The Dental Advisor.* "You want staffers who make learning a personal and professional priority—and who consider CE part of their total compensation package. Be frank about your view of the responsibilities for and rewards of CE, and insist on frankness in return. Explain your practice culture and ask questions such as:

"How do your goals fit in with our practice vision?"

"What goals have you recently pursued?"

"What's the most valuable CE experience you've ever had?"

"If someone doesn't show interest in these questions," says the *Dental Practice Advisor* "or flatly states he or she doesn't care one way or the other—recognize that he or she will consider CE an *obligation*, not a benefit. At best, attendance will be half-hearted. At worst, that person will fight you or find excuses to actively avoid CE opportunities."[21]

HARD-LEARNED LESSON

"Our behavior is driven by a fundamental core belief: the desire and the ability of an organization to continuously learn from any source, anywhere—and to rapidly convert this learning into action is its ultimate competitive advantage" (Jack Welch, former CEO of General Electric).[22]

---

157 Ask behavior-based questions

Behavior-based questions require job applicants to reveal specific information about how they handled particular situations in the past. The purpose is to predict a person's *future performance* based on his or her *past job experience*. The following questions are some examples:

- "In your previous job(s), were you ever asked to stay late on a day when you had other plans? What did you do and how did you feel about it?"
- "Describe a time when you encountered obstacles in your last job while you were in pursuit of a goal. What happened?"
- "Describe a situation that occurred in your last job that required great patience on your part. How did you deal with it?"
- "Have you ever had to deal with an irate patient (customer, client)? What happened?"
- "Have you ever had to deal with coworkers who didn't cooperate or contribute a fair share of the work? What did you do in those situations?"

"Behavioral interviewing does not replace the need to evaluate the technical skills and qualifications of candidates," say Lawrence H. Stone, DDS, MAGD, ABGD, Doylestown, PA, and consultant Scott Drinnan, Philadelphia, PA. "What it does is provide an additional dimension that expands what you can learn beyond traditional interviewing techniques."[23]

REALITY CHECK
As revealing as the replies to such questions might be in evaluating a job applicant, not all candidates are going to be comfortable in answering them. Use such questions sparingly and move on to other matters as the situation warrants.

158 Check out the person's "view of the world"

"Nothing better indicates a candidate's confidence than his or her view of the world in general," writes Robert Half, President of the recruiting firm Robert Half International, Inc. "Are they optimistic or pessimistic?" he asks. "Do they view the proverbial glass as half empty or half full? People with a positive viewpoint are infinitely more likely to be happier, more productive and more efficient. They are easier to motivate, quicker to learn and adapt to a variety of situations, and in general, have greater potential to become top-notch employees."

When evaluating competing candidates for a job, Half recommends that when all else is equal, chose the person who most wants the job.[24]

159 Hard-learned lessons about hiring

Jack Welch, former chairman and CEO of General Electric, claims that 90% of good management is about getting the right people in the right jobs.[25]

Every employee contributes to a patient's impression of your office—for better or for worse.

"Staff accounts for 60 to 80 percent of the overall image of a practice and a patient's decision about whether to return," says Clarksville, TN, consultant Ronald E. Whitford, DVM.

Don't rely on first impressions. Many dentists and office managers make up their minds about an applicant within the first few minutes. It can be a huge mistake. You can miss the real person.

If a new employee doesn't have the right attitude about work or the right personality for your practice, it's unlikely a written script of what to say to patients or even on-the-job training is going to make a difference.

"Staff your company," says author Ron Zemke, "with people who don't see their jobs as burdens and chores. Look for individuals who get a kick out of serving other people. Look for employees who find customer contact exciting and rewarding—who don't find any aspect of serving others demeaning. They're the ones who will deliver service that will set your business apart."[26]

Be careful not to mistake a quiet, reserved demeanor for a lack of motivation.

Be careful also not to mistake a person's ability to play the "interview game," or his or her ability to talk easily, for intelligence or competence.

"Please give me an example." These are the five most important words in the interviewer's arsenal and they can't be used enough. There is nothing worse than ending an interview and finding an extraordinary comment in your notes for which there is not a shred of supporting evidence.

Beware of wishful thinking. It arises because of a desperate need to hire someone and as a result leads you to overlook traits that under different circumstances would disqualify the job applicant. Remind yourself of the costs and aggravation involved in a bad hire.

Don't oversell a job by promising more than you can deliver or, conversely, by downplaying the negative aspects of a job. When the facts become known, a new employee will either become demotivated or quit. Face the facts: *a job is what it is.* One solution: rethink the position. Can the appealing aspects of the job be broadened? Can less desirable aspects be traded or possibly divided among other employees, perhaps outsourced?

"Pay attention to the final five minutes," says Steven L. Rasner, DDS, Cherry Hill, NJ. "Announce casually that 'We're just about out of time.' Many candidates will save their most important comments or questions until the very end, so give them the chance," he says, "to help you see what's important. You may hear a question such as 'Do we ever have to work weekends or overtime?' The closing minutes can offer the clearest insights to your candidate's concerns."[27]

Always ask job applicants, "What am I likely to hear, positive and negative, when I call your references?" The question gives them an opportunity to brag about their previous job strengths and achievements. It also enables them to tell their side of any negative story you might hear (or one they *think* you might hear).

Never hire someone whose first question is, "What are the benefits?"

Never hire someone you can't fire, such as friends and relatives.

As certain as you might be that you've found the perfect candidate, resist the temptation to hire somebody on the spot, unless you've been unable to fill the job for a long time and delay could jeopardize your chances of hiring the person. In general, it's always good to give yourself a day or two to make sure you're not overlooking faults that could later surface. The best approach: let the candidate know you're interested and ask for a day or two to make the final decision.

Don't ignore intuition. As objective as hiring needs to be, one should not ignore that "tug" inside that says "something just doesn't feel right here." Often this comes from your past experience and facts you've had to face through the years. Listen to that inner voice.

Notes

1. Bonner P. The Importance of Staff, *Dentistry Today,* July 2004, 8.
2. Deal TE, Kennedy AA. Corporate Cultures: *The Rites and Rituals of Corporate Life*. Reading MA: Addison-Wesley, 1982.
3. Wilde JA. *How Dentistry Can Be a Joyous Path to Financial Freedom*. Hamilton, IL: The Novel Pen, 1996.
4. Williams C. *Management*. Stamford, CT, Southwestern College Publishing, 2000.
5. *Journal of the American Compensation Association,* Winter 1995.
6. Sunoo BP. Results-Oriented Customer Service Training. *Workforce,* May 2001, 84-90.
7. James KR. Ask the Expert: How Can I Find the Right Employee? *Journal of the American Dental Association,* July 1999, 1101-1103.
8. Rasner SL. Hire Right. *Dental Practice Report,* October 2000, 37-44.
9. Dickerson WG. Frontdesklessness and the Quality Practice. *Dentistry Today,* March 1993, 82-85.
10. Freiberg K, Freiberg J. *Nuts! Southwest Airlines' Crazy Recipe for Business and Personal Success*. Austin, TX: Bard Press, 1996.
11. The First Words in Personnel Management: Careful Hiring, *Blair/McGill Advisory,* August 1995, 4.
12. Booth N. Hire for Attitude, Train for Skill. *Dental Economics,* October 2000, 85-89.
13. Kiger PJ. Why Customer Satisfaction Starts With HR. *Workforce,* May 2002, 26-32.
14. Miller C. Interviewing Dos and Don'ts. *AGD Impact,* March 2004, 16-17.
15. Pride JR. In Search of Your Ideal Employee. *Dental Practice Report,* May/June 1999.
16. Blair CW. How Top Practices Reduce Labor Costs. *Blair/McGill Advisory,* April 1998, 3-4.
17. Thompson CB. *Recruit by Targeting the Right Employees,* Frankfort, IL: Training Systems.
18. Pride JR, Morgan A. The Many Hats of Dentistry. *Dental Economics,* September 2003, 58-64, 150.
19. Moin K. Five Ways to Make Your Web Site a Profitbuilder. *Blair/McGill Advisory,* July 2003, 4.

20. Black A. Benefits: Money Well Spent? *Review of Optometry,* June 2001, 37.
21. Gutter SA, Hammond JE, Laring A, et al. Discuss Staff CE Expectations Before Hiring, *Dental Practice Advisor,* October 2000, 7.
22. Krames JA. *Exceptional Leaders and Their Lessons for Transforming any Business.* New York: McGraw-Hill, 2003.
23. Stone LH, Drinnan S. The Behavioral Interview in Dentistry. *Dental Economics,* October 2003, 138-143.
24. Half R. *Finding, Hiring, and Keeping the Best Employees.* New York: John Wiley & Sons, 1993.
25. Nelson B. Self-Motivation, Fact or Fiction. *Corporate Meetings & Incentives,* December 2001, 45.
26. Zemke R. Secrets of Knock Your Socks-Off Service. *Bottom Line Business,* April 1998.
27. Rasner SL. Hire Right, *Dental Practice Report,* October 2000, 37-44.

12

Be an "Employer of Choice"

The war for top talent has become fierce. As the need for well-qualified, high-performing employees intensifies, employers vie to position themselves as the right place for the kind of people they want. They strive to become known as an "Employer of Choice."

High-performance dental practices are typically Employers of Choice. They tend to have higher levels of staff morale, motivation, and productivity; less absenteeism and turnover; enhanced loyalty; more efficiency and, as a result, greater profitability.

Dentists/Employers of Choice are also more attractive to patients. This appeal is critical in a relationship-based environment. Patients like to deal with the same people on a long-term basis. This relationship continuity builds stronger bonds and gives patients a greater sense of comfort, confidence, and trust.

REALITY CHECK

Dentists/Employers of Choice are by definition more attractive to prospective employees. Not only do they have more applicants to choose from, but the overall quality of applicants tends to be better than for practices that are not recognized as Employers of Choice.

This chapter and Chapters 13 and 14 will include the major steps in becoming an Employer of Choice.

160 Build your "employment brand"

Employment branding has been described as the process of developing a reputation as a "great place to work" (i.e., Employer of Choice) in the minds of those you'd like to hire for your practice. It is similar to the concept of branding your practice as described in Chapter 3.

Your employment brand is an essential, invaluable commodity in a tight labor market. It's what people say about your practice when they're with their friends and describe what it's like to work there. If your practice has a positive brand image, job applicants will be predisposed in favor of your practice. They'll immediately know your name and reputation as a dentist and as an "Employer of Choice."

FROM THE SUCCESS FILES

"Even before her interview, Doris Barnett had a good feeling about Dr. Jim Kaley's practice," says Laura Pelehach, managing editor of *Dental Practice Report*. "The ad in the paper stressed a fun work environment and good benefits. She liked that, but even more, she liked what she had been hearing about the Greensboro, North Carolina, orthodontist's practice."

"'I was told that you either have to wait until someone dies or moves away before you have a chance of working there,' says Barnett, a former insurance company secretary and one of 40 candidates vying for the secretarial spot."

"On the rare occasion when he is in the market to hire, Kaley generally has his pick of quality employees. He has a reputation in his community as a good orthodontist and good employer, which appeals to candidates like Barnett. But the truth of the matter is, he doesn't often have to worry about hiring. Most of Kaley's employees have been there at least 10 years, some for almost 25 of the 29 years Kaley has been practicing. He likes his staff."

"That's no small feat," says Pelehach, "considering many dentists still grapple with high turnover."[1]

HARD-LEARNED LESSON

"Having a strong brand for employees is a competitive advantage and a strategic advantage," says. Beth Sawi, chief administrative officer, Charles Schwab. "It really does help us attract the best candidates."[2]

161 Get them off to the right start

"How new employees are treated on their first day," writes James B. Miller, author of *The Corporate Coach*, "makes an indelible impression that affects long-term performance. Quite frankly," he adds, "it is the most important day in an employee's career. It sets the tone for everything that will follow. How employees are treated on their first day is something every manager should make a top priority."[3]

Regardless of a person's work history, a staff member's first day on a new job can be intimidating. For some, it is so overwhelming and confusing that they don't return for a second day.

The following guidelines may help make the transition for new employees a smoother, more positive experience.

Send a "Welcome to the Practice" letter to the homes of new employees *before* their first day. It lets them (and their families) know they're important members of a healthcare team and that you're looking forward to working together.

On the first day, pair the new staff member with a co-worker who will serve as a coach and encouraging presence for as long as needed. This has two advantages. First, it gives a new staff member a one-on-one way to "learn the ropes" from someone who's been in his or her shoes. Second, the coach feels proud you chose him or her to be personally responsible for the new team member. A coach can be any staff member who's had a couple years of experience at your practice, exhibits leadership qualities, and wants to help new employees grow in their jobs

If possible, avoid starting a new employee on the busiest day of the week. For most practices, it's better to start on a Tuesday or Wednesday than on a Monday or Friday.

Make sure to let all staff members know that the new employee is expected and ask them to make him or her feel welcome.

The orientation should include a thorough review of the employee handbook. You want new employees familiar with your policies and to have all work-related questions answered.

During the orientation and/or initial training phase, be attuned to a new person's need for information and individual capacity for learning. Some new employees may want to move quickly beyond the basics to learn about the broader issues such as the core values and philosophy of the practice.

During the break-in period, the coach can monitor the new staff member's progress with such questions as "Do you have the resources you need to do the job?" "Do you need any assistance in dealing with anyone in the practice?" "Is the job what you expected it would be?" "Is there anything we can do for you?"

New employees should finish their first day feeling they've made the right decision and joined the type of practice for which they want to work.

REALITY CHECK

Finally and perhaps most important, you must decide that welcoming a new staff member is an investment in long-term retention and should be given a high priority.

162 Make work enjoyable

By making work enjoyable, says consultant Matt Weinstein, PhD, you help create the kind of organization to which your employees will want to make a long-term commitment and where turnover and burnout will be minimal. The intentional use of fun, he adds, can have an enormous impact on team building, stress management, employee morale, and the way patients are treated.[4]

FROM THE SUCCESS FILES

"There's no more powerful, positive emotion than laughter," says Ken Snyder, DMD, Phoenix, AZ. "We look better, feel better, perform better, and are more productive and creative when we are happy. Now here's the key," he adds, "for years it was thought we laugh because we are happy, but now it's believed we are actually happy because we laugh. We dentists," Dr. Snyder adds, "need to take our profession seriously, but not ourselves so seriously."[5]

Does this sound appealing? From the success files of high-performance practices, here are some ideas to generate a sense of fun in an office.

- "Give yourself and your staff permission to have fun with each other and with patients," says consultant/author Paul Homoly, DDS, Holt, MI.[6]
- Let people bring homegrown, homemade, or store-bought food to work on a rotating basis. Snack food is fun and promotes camaraderie. Establish a budget for the purpose.
- Even better, contract with a local produce distributor to supply your office with fresh fruit when in season. A fruit snack is a healthy treat and energy-boosting alternative to coffee-break foods. Start with once a week to see how it goes. An added benefit: it will make employees feel they're special and they work in a special place.
- Place a dry erase board in a central location where anyone (doctors or staff members) can write a compliment or thank you to anyone else.
- Have in-office lunches, catered or otherwise. These are great for staff meetings, celebrations, and bad-weather days.
- Fresh flowers, from the garden or delivered by a florist, are always uplifting and well worth the investment.
- Have a staff lounge where employees can take a break, renew their spirits, have a snack or a group luncheon, or simply let their hair down. Decorate with humorous posters, cartoons, and anti-stress toys. A microwave oven is a must. Exercise equipment is another option.
- Have parties for employee birthdays, anniversaries, going away or "welcome aboard" occasions or, perhaps, for no reason at all. Make these festive occasions. Consider flowers or balloons, coffee and cake, perhaps a catered lunch. Exchange gag gifts.

FROM THE SUCCESS FILES

At his practice's year-end holiday party, Chris Kammer, DDS, president and owner of the Center for Cosmetic Dentistry in Madison, WI, had a surprise for his staff of 25. When the employees finished eating, he asked them to wait a few minutes. Then two stretch limousines driven by chauffeurs in Santa outfits pulled up to the curb outside the office. The staff was invited to climb into the limos and drink champagne, eat bonbons, and sing along to a holiday CD that Dr. Kammer himself had burned.

The employees were whisked to a local mall, where he presented each of them with a $100 bill and gave them an hour to spend it all. Whatever money they didn't spend in that time, they had to return.

While the main reward was still money, Dr. Kammer said he believed that the experience surrounding it would be more fondly remembered than the cash of years past.

"The money alone was drab," he said. "This is something they're never going to forget."[7]

You don't have to be elaborate. Fun activities need only provide a change of pace, a way to unwind if only for a few minutes, a way to celebrate and appreciate each other.

The mood of a practice is important. If your practice is an upbeat place to be, your patients will pick up on it, and you and your staff will be better for it.

---

163 Encourage upward communication

The fact that you never hear job-related complaints from employees doesn't necessarily mean everyone is happy. Many employees are reluctant to speak up when they dislike something about their work or the way they're treated by their boss. Some are timid or afraid. Others think speaking up would be a waste of time because nothing would change if they did. So they talk among themselves and their families, perhaps with patients as well, about the things that bother them about the practice. And the problems continue.

Eventually this lack of communication takes its toll. Unhappy people do not perform as well as those who like their jobs. They're not as interested in what they do or how well they do it. They tend to be slower, perhaps more careless, and they're not as pleasant. In time, it begins to affect everyone's morale, patients included.

Firing unhappy employees isn't the answer. Effective management and motivation of people depend on good communication—*upward* as well as downward.

Downward communication takes place when the doctor does the talking and the staff listens. Upward communication is the just the opposite. The staff talks. The *doctor* listens.

REALITY CHECK
"After more than 40 years in business," says J.W. Marriott, chairman and CEO of Marriott International, Inc., "I've concluded that listening

is the single most important on-the-job skill that a good manager can cultivate. A leader who doesn't listen well risks missing critical information, losing (or never winning) the confidence of staff and peers, and forfeiting the opportunity to be a proactive, hands-on manager."[8]

Upward communication is the only way dentists can ascertain the level of staff morale and job satisfaction and what changes, if any, are needed to improve them. It's also the key to discovering what impact their management style has on others.

Upward communication is only meaningful if employees are free to "tell it like it is," and confident the doctor will listen with an open mind. If they're concerned their job security or future raises might in any way be threatened by what they say, it's understandable (and predictable) they'll say only what they think the doctor *wants* to hear. And the problems will continue.

164 A simple prescription

"This is a simple prescription that can help solve a multitude of morale problems," says practice management consultant/speaker Bill Rossi. "Simply make a point of spending 15 to 25 minutes one-on-one with each staff member over the course of the next three weeks. Go out for a cup of coffee or take a walk around the block—someplace where you can visit with the person quietly and confidentially. As practice management lecturer Dr. Ken James suggests, ask each team member the following three questions:

"How are you doing?"

"How am I doing?"

"How are we doing?"

"At first," Rossi says, "you may not get much of an answer, but let the silence be and your staff will be forthcoming. If staff members make statements or complaints that you believe are unjustified, do not comment or try to defend yourself. Instead, simply listen and at the end of the meeting, look the person in the eye and say, 'I will take what you say under consideration.' And then do that."

"The act of just meeting with staff members individually," says Dr. Rossi, "can be therapeutic. By venting their feelings, employees are often able to overcome their hostilities and become re-involved in the practice. It's a simple and effective prescription to begin to make things better."[9]

165 The employee survey

Another more comprehensive technique for initiating upward communication is the employee survey. It's widely used as a management tool in industry to learn what employees think of their jobs, working conditions, quality of supervision, compensation, co-workers, opportunities for advancement and other factors.

The advantage of the employee survey is that many employees are more comfortable expressing themselves *anonymously* on paper than they are in person. This greatly improves the chances of getting truthful results.

The following is a composite of employee surveys used in a wide variety of healthcare professions. Use or modify for your particular situation. Add additional questions. And leave space for employees to elaborate on their answers.

Employee Survey

	Strongly Agree	Agree	Strongly Disagree	Disagree

1) The people I work with help each other out when someone falls behind or gets in a tight spot.

2) When changes are made that affect me, I am usually told the reasons for the changes.

3) The doctor really tries to get our ideas about things.

4) The doctor's review of my performance gives me a clear picture of how I'm doing on the job.

5) The practice could benefit from more frequent staff meetings.

6) My job is a satisfactory challenge to me.

7) Our staff meetings are a waste of time.

8) If I have a complaint, I feel free to tell the doctor about it.

9) The doctor has always been fair in dealing with me.

10) I look forward to coming to work.

11) The doctor lets us know exactly what's expected of us.

12) There's too much pressure in my job.

13) Some of the working conditions here need to be changed.

14) I'm paid fairly compared with other employees.

15) My job has not turned out to be as it was described to me when I was hired.

16) I have all the authority I need to perform my job properly.

17) I have been properly trained to do my job.

18) I am very much underpaid for the work I do.

19) I have the right equipment and materials to do my job well.

20) The office policies are clearly spelled out.

21) I am given the opportunity to learn and grow in my job.

22) I feel my efforts to do a good job are appreciated.

23) I enjoy working with the people here.

24) The doctor lets me know in a fair and constructive manner when I have done something wrong.

25) The hours of work are satisfactory.

26) Our productivity sometimes suffers from lack of organization and planning.

27) I think some good may come out of completing this survey.

Optional: The reason I feel as I do about question # _____ is: _____

What I think should be done about it is: _____

REALITY CHECK

Will such a survey open a can of worms? Create more problems than it solves? The answer is "no." Problems either do or do not already exist. Ignoring them won't make them go away. It may in fact, make them *worse*, lead to deep resentment, and cause a capable person to quit.

Evidence indicates that the attitude of employees tends to improve when they're given an opportunity to speak their minds. It's why such surveys are so widely used in industry.

166 The problem that has no name

"We live in a culture, especially at work, that prefers harmony over discord, agreement over dissent, speed over deliberation," says Leslie A. Perlow, associate professor at the Harvard Business School. "Whether with colleagues, friends, or family members, the tendency to paper over differences rather than confront them is extremely common. We believe the best thing to preserve our relationships and to ensure our work gets done as expeditiously as possible is to silence conflict." She dubs it: "the problem that has no name."[10]

Dental practices are not immune to what Ms. Perlow calls "the vicious spiral of silence." Examples include team members who stifle their feelings about being underpaid or underappreciated or who are bored by their work. Dentists, too, have their reasons for failing to confront employees who are often late for work or who are careless about keeping the office spotlessly clean or perhaps socialize too much with patients.

"If no one expresses their thoughts," Ms. Perlow writes, "people will likely continue thinking and behaving in the same way and nothing will change. Problems are likely to persist and may even get worse because corrective actions are not taken."

One of the costs of silencing conflict, Ms. Perlow says, is the effect it has on employee motivation and engagement. When work relationships are marked by pent-up frustration, our work suffers and it is hard to be motivated as a result. "We don't experience a reason to put much of ourselves into our job, be creative or go above and beyond the call of duty. Instead we may lose interest in our work and start to disengage from it and our organization–psychologically, at first, and then often physically, by quitting. This is highly costly for both individuals and organizations."

ACTION STEPS
The best advice for anyone caught in this bind, advises Ms. Perlow, is to speak up and seek mutual understanding. Employee surveys and performance reviews (see Chapter 13) are two ways to start the process. Talking things over may not solve all the problems. It may, however, clarify them; enable you to learn each other's needs; make needed adjustments; and improve the productivity of your practice.

FROM THE SUCCESS FILES
Keeping the lines of communication open is essential to being a good manager. Sam Platia, administrator of the five-clinician Northwestern Medical Center in New Tripoli, PA, says he periodically meets with employees and asks for their ideas and how their jobs can be modified. "They know their jobs better than anyone," he says. "Feedback from them and making them feel part of a team increases the likelihood of a successful staff and smooth-running practice."[11]

167 The subtle influence of employees

"Employees, of course, have the greatest impact in their dealings with customers," says The Wall Street Journal editor/writer Ronald J. Alsop. "As many companies know all too well, poor service does incredible damage to their reputations. But what many companies underestimate is the more subtle influence of employees—from the executive suite to the mailroom—on reputation. Employees' behavior and comments outside business hours can carry significant weight. They affect how their friends, neighbors, and relatives feel about the company. In many cases, people's only experience with a company is through its employees. Word-of-mouth impressions gleaned from employees can be quite positive if they're fiercely loyal to their companies—or deadly if they're miserable in their jobs."[12]

168 Employees are #1

HARD-LEARNED LESSON

Don't cave in to patients who abuse, insult, and intimidate your employees. Recognize the incredibly deflating message it sends employees if you side with an abusive patient while ignoring the rights and dignity of your own staff.

FROM THE SUCCESS FILES

"Step in at the appropriate moment with the appropriate support," says Tom Orent, DMD, Framingham, MA. "Give your team the authority to tell you that this patient makes them too uncomfortable—and that the patient should be asked to leave the practice. Our team members have always had this right," he adds, "and have very rarely used it."[13]

Imagine the level of commitment that emanates from such a willingness to dismiss a patient who hassles a member of your staff.

Dentists who have taken this step tell me they get a variety of actions. Some of these patients realize they've been out of line, apologize for their behavior, and become model citizens. Others take the hint and leave.

As a speaker, I've asked countless audiences of dentists and staff members if anyone has ever *regretted* dismissing patients who were disruptive or troublesome in some other way. Examples include those who Rudy Dunnigan, DMD, Ashland, KY, labels "high-maintenance patients who require excessive attention; chronic complainers who always find something to gripe about; and patients with high expectations and low compliance."[14]

The only regret I've heard (and it's expressed frequently) is, "I wish we had done it *sooner*."

ACTION STEP

"Do yourself and your patients a favor," says James H. Hastings, DDS, Placerville, CA. "Politely dismiss those patients who create stress for you and your staff. These patients distract you from giving 100 percent to patients who appreciate your services."[15]

REALITY CHECK

Lawyers advise that you should check with your malpractice insurer before taking any steps related to dismissing a patient. There are important issues regarding abandonment that need to be considered—including those that exist within the confines of a managed care plan's provider panel.

Resource. The American Dental Association has a booklet entitled *Terminating the Dentist-Patient Relationship: Questions and Answers* (item L 204). It can be ordered from their Web site at www.adacatalog.org or by telephone at 1-800-947-4746.

169 Celebrate!

"Do you know why most employees leave their jobs?" asks Lawrence Ragan Communications, Inc. "Because they get in a 'rut' and are, in a word, bored. Sweep employees out of their ruts by launching 'guerilla celebration' attacks. Close the office for one hour on Friday morning to have a 'comedy party' where you show videos of popular sitcoms. Announce on Monday that Friday will be a half-day, for no reason. Have bagels and coffee waiting for employees on a random Tuesday. Keep employees off balance about what you're going to do next. It's the sort of thing that separates one company from another—and convinces employees to stay put when they are thinking about leaving."[16]

Whether or not you want to go to these lengths, there's no denying that celebrations with plenty of public pats on the back are a great way to make your staff feel like they're on a winning team. What can you celebrate? Ask your staff for ideas. The following is a short list of possibilities:

- The achievement of practice goals.
- Your practice's anniversary.
- The 100th (or 1000th) completion of a given procedure.
- The busiest day, week, or month since the beginning of the year.
- To mark the end of a project or major effort such as a new computer, a practice Web site, a major change in appointment scheduling, eliminating insurance, or achieving "front desklessness."

From the Success Files

"The best tool you can have is a great staff," says William Dorfman, DDS, Beverly Hills, CA. "If they are not great, replace them. Mediocrity isn't going to make it in our profession. Following the construction and our move into a modern, new suite, I took my staff out to dinner. I had hired three new people who work up front in addition to the three I had before. It is a big staff, and they were doing an amazing job. They love their work. They are friendly. My office has never run more efficiently. Just in appreciation of that, I said, 'Let's all go out to dinner tonight.' And I took the whole staff out for a really nice dinner."

"I can't do what I do without them."[17]

HARD-LEARNED LESSON

When things go well in your practice, make a point of celebrating the victory and the people who made it possible. Recognize and thank everyone involved for his or her efforts. It will nourish team spirit. Make people proud to be part of your practice. Burnish your reputation as an Employer of Choice.

Notes

1. Pelehach L. Today's Employees Are Changing . . . Are You? *Dental Practice Report,* November 2001, 18-24.
2. Engaging Employees Through Your Brand. *The Conference Board,* Research Report 1288-01-ES, 2001.
3. Miller JB. *The Corporate Coach.* New York: HarperBusiness, 1993.
4. Weinstein M. *Managing to Have Fun at Work.* New York: Simon & Schuster, 1996.
5. Snyder K. A Chuckle a Day Keeps the Doctor Away. *Dental Management,* June 1991, 43-45.
6. Homoly P. Opportunity Knocks. *Dental Economics,* August 2001.
7. Ligos M. Those Year-End Bonuses Aren't Always Green. *The New York Times,* December 28, 2003, BU 8.
8. Marriott JW, Jr., Brown KA. *The Spirit to Serve.* New York: HarperBusiness, 1997.
9. Rossi B. How to Reinvigorate a Jaded Staff. *Dental Practice & Finance,* July/August 1997, 14-19.
10. Perlow LA. *When You Say Yes But Mean No.* New York: Crown Business, 2003.
11. Weiss GG. Turn a Problem Employee into a Pearl. *Medical Economics,* December 2002, 19-25.
12. Alsop RJ. *The 18 Immutable Laws of Corporate Reputation.* New York: Free Press, 2004.
13. Orent T. Academy Gems. *AACD Journal,* Fall 1996, 36.
14. Dunnigan R. Stop and Smell the Eugenol! *Dental Economics,* January 2003, 14-18.
15. Allen J. Shortening the Learning Curve. *AACD Journal,* Winter 1997, 49-55.
16. www.ragan.com, accessed 9/4/04.
17. Clinician's Comments. *Dental Products Report,* May 1997, 66-70.

13

Secrets of Staff Retention

Let's start with a few obvious but troubling facts. Employee turnover is expensive. Finding new talent is challenging. Training new people is time consuming. Retaining employees once they have gained experience and expertise at your expense continues to be difficult.

Low levels of employee satisfaction threaten staff morale, patient relations, and practice growth and, in turn, lead to profit-draining high turnover rates.

170 The high cost of turnover

To calculate your annual employee turnover rate, divide this year's number of employee defections by the total number of staff, and then multiply by 100. If the staff turnover rate exceeds 15% on average during the last 5 years, your practice is considered to have high turnover, says California consultant Judy Capko.[1]

Employee replacement costs are estimated at 25% of annual compensation, including the costs of recruitment, training, and the time a new employee takes to reach his or her maximum efficiency level. Turnover also takes a huge toll on staff morale and patient satisfaction. Thus focusing your attention on improving staff retention rates can accomplish much more than just improving your bottom line.

REALITY CHECK

The average tenure of a worker at a given job is 3.6 years, according to the U.S. Bureau of Labor Statistics.[2]

171   Ask for commitment, not loyalty

"At Brush-Wellman Inc., we are asking for the commitment—not loyalty of employees," says Daniel Skoch, vice president of human resources. "Commitment requires an agreement to do something; loyalty implies being blindly faithful to a duty or obligation. Thus we have begun to tell our employees:

'We will help you grow and develop. We will provide you opportunities to learn, to be involved, to practice new skills, to have responsibility, to be respected and valued, and to be rewarded and recognized for your contributions. In return, we seek your commitment to our company's mission. We cannot guarantee what is going to happen in the future, but if it doesn't work out, you will leave here a more talented, responsible, self-confident and employable person.'"

"As a result," says Mr. Skoch, "we believe that our employees recognize that their personal needs for security, growth opportunities, and job satisfaction can link up very well with the company's need for employees who are willing to continually learn, and be adaptable and self-supervising. This linking will provide us with a competitive advantage and our employees with their best opportunity for personal security."[3]

172   Do your employees realize how much they're paid?

Many dental staff members I've interviewed look at their compensation strictly in terms of *take-home pay*, without considering the substantial *fringe benefits* they also receive. Knowing all the facts makes employees realize how much they're actually paid and often has an immediate and highly positive impact on morale, motivation, and staff retention.

To make employees aware of the total compensation they receive, provide them annually with a *year-end benefits statement* (an example is given in the box that follows) with their W-2 form. List the dollar value of the many extras your practice offers that otherwise may be overlooked or taken for granted.

Year-End Benefits Statement

This statement is a summary of the various forms of compensation you receive as a staff member of this practice.

Benefit	**Value ($)**
Gross base salary	
Overtime and bonuses	
Health insurance premium (for employee and dependents)	
Pension/profit sharing plan	
Employer's contribution to Social Security	
State unemployment insurance premium	
Workers' compensation insurance premium	
Discounted professional services	
Paid holidays	
Paid vacations	
Sick leave	
Uniform allowance	
Continuing education costs (tuition, transportation, lodging, and meals)	
Professional dues and subscriptions	
Other	

Delete those benefits that are not applicable and add others such as 401K plan benefits if they are part of an employee's salary package. Then add the *total dollar value* of each employee's salary and benefits. In most cases, it will be substantially higher than the person's take-home pay.

The problem often is that many employees simply don't know what they're getting. The year-end benefits statement is meant to close that gap. It's also an excellent tool for employee recruitment and retention.

173 Equity theory

Equity theory states that when employees feel underpaid, they will find a way to rectify the situation. The most obvious ways are to quit or ask for a raise. Other more devious ways include attempts to make one's job more rewarding in *nonfinancial ways* such as socializing with co-workers, taking long breaks, or making personal phone calls. These attempts may include slowing down at work, taking more sick leave, or becoming less attentive to details. (Telltale sign: three people are needed to do the job of two.) If feelings run deeper, the attempts may result in "white collar crime" such as stealing, just to "even the score."

According to equity theory, employees compare what's called their *job inputs* (education, skills, experience, responsibility, productivity, years on the job) and *job outputs* (salary and benefits) with *those of co-workers.* When this ratio is out of balance, a sense of *inequity* is experienced. It happens, for example, when an employee thinks his or her job is more difficult or demanding than that of a coworker who's paid the same, let alone a *higher,* salary.

ACTION STEPS

"The lack of *written job descriptions* often results in some employees doing more (or less) than they were initially hired to do," says David Goodnight DVM, MBA, consultant, Dallas, TX. "For a variety of reasons," he adds, "it just happens and in time, the overworked person is likely to sense an inequity. The solution is to adjust workloads, salaries, or benefits and if necessary, hire additional people—even if it means increasing overhead. In the end, you'll have greatly improved employee morale, productivity, and practice growth."

REALITY CHECK

"The degree of active behavior that under-rewarded employees will take is largely dependent on how equity-sensitive they are," says Stephen P. Robbins, PhD, faculty member (emeritus) at San Diego State University. "Some employees are very good at ignoring inequities or adjusting their perceptions to make them less bothersome. But many professional and technical employees are equity-sensitive. They're likely to move quickly to correct any perceived inequity."[4]

174 Performance reviews

Studies show that a high percentage of employees are in the dark about how they're doing on the job or how they can do better, simply because they've never been told and have no way of knowing.

One result is that exceptional employees are unaware of their strengths and may or may not be consistent in what they do or how they do it. Those who feel their efforts are unnoticed and unappreciated may become demotivated or, worse, start looking for another job.

Another result is that marginal employees are unaware of their shortcomings, and may assume that silence means approval (i.e., "If the doctor didn't like the way I do things, he would tell me.")

Either way, you lose.

One solution to this communication gap is the *performance review*. It's been defined as a two-way dialogue between employer and employee about the latter's past, present, and future job performance. It includes a discussion of such matters as the following:

- Recognition of good work.
- Clarification of job responsibilities and priorities.
- Suggestions for improvement on both sides.
- Agreement on how and by when such improvements will be made.

Such discussions let people know how their performance on the job compares with your expectations. This understanding helps employees identify their strengths, develop their talents, and enjoy their work.

Note. Many dentists avoid performance reviews because of the concern they'll be asked for a raise. The fact is that *salary reviews* and *performance reviews* are separate and distinct management tasks and should be scheduled at different times.

ACTION STEPS

Schedule a performance review in advance and give employees a list of those topics and/or questions (such as the following) that are most appropriate for their situation. It will give them time to think about the issues that concern them.

Before you discuss the person, discuss the job itself. You may have different ideas about the exact nature of each job than your employees do. If you have a written job description, review it together to see if it needs revision. Then ask such questions as:

- "Do we agree on what your job is?"
- "Which do you think are the most important elements of your job? Do we agree on these?"
- "Do we agree on the standards by which your work will be evaluated?"

Ask Before You Tell. Instead of *telling* employees what you think of their work, *ask* them (individually) to tell you what they think they have done well and what they would like to do better. Many will criticize themselves more readily than they will accept criticism from you. In fact, they may judge themselves more harshly than you would. The following questions may help facilitate the discussion:

- "What do you think are your greatest strengths?"
- "In which areas do you feel less competent?"
- "Do you feel you are becoming more competent as time goes by? If so, in what ways?"
- "What could we do to help you do your job better?"
- "Do I do anything that makes your job harder?"

Management expert Peter Drucker says, "The greatest boost to productivity would be for managers to ask, 'What do we do in this organization that helps you do the job you're being paid for—and what do we do that hampers you?'"

Keep Criticism Impersonal by Discussing "Job performance" Only. For example, you can call a person "irresponsible" or you can say, "This job was to be completed by the 15th and it wasn't done until the 18th." The first statement is opinion and open to question. The second is fact.

Determine the Cause of Poor Performance. Encourage employees to analyze problems by asking, "That's an unusual number of billing errors. What happened?" or "How can we prevent this from happening in the future?" Then wait for an answer.

Don't Get Bogged Down in Finding Fault. The problem with evaluations is dwelling on what's wrong and how to fix it rather than what's right and how to make it better. Conclude by discussing a particular strength and how to build on it (see secret #175).

Agree on a Plan of Action. The improvement you want in an employee's work habits or performance can occur only when you both perceive the problem in the same way and agree on both the means and a timetable for solving it.

Start with Your Recommendations, or better yet, invite your employees to tell you how they would like to develop themselves and what help, if any, they would like from you. Be specific. Set deadlines. Then put this "action plan" on paper as a form of "contract" between you and your employee. Each of you should have a copy. Such commitment will get better results than vague promises. The action plan will also serve as a benchmark against which future progress (or, if necessary, grounds for dismissal) can be measured.

REALITY CHECK

"When performance changes are requested of an employee," says consultant/speaker Julie H. Weir, "there are three questions that the dentist can ask to get insight into whether or not the employee will be successful. Ask 'Is this a change you want to make?' 'Is this a change you think you can make?' and 'What kind of help do you need to make this change?'"[5]

175 Focus on strengths

When conducting performance reviews, don't dwell on an employee's shortcomings. There's no faster way to put people off than to criticize them, even if the criticism is given under the guise of "performance evaluation."

Instead, talk to their strengths. Start by observing people's everyday behavior in broad categories and then get more specific.

How attentive to detail is the person? Is he or she especially good with children? Older people?

Is the person cheerful, friendly, caring, creative, diplomatic, willing to help others, kind, enthusiastic, hard-working, a good listener, funny, intelligent, interesting, open-minded, well-organized, patient, upbeat, punctual, polite, sensitive, self-starting, thoughtful, unselfish, versatile?

These are only a few of the positive characteristics you or an office manager can reflect back to a team member at a performance review or anytime, for that matter.

The dentist or office manager who only addresses his or her people's strengths at performance reviews is missing opportunities on every other working day to boost morale and productivity.

If you'll look for and share one positive strength in a staff member per day, no matter how minuscule, the boost to that individual's morale and performance will be astounding.

REALITY CHECK

When employees are hired, they bring with them a vast array of strengths developed from their previous education, work experiences, avocational pursuits, civic or charity organizational work, and the like that, in many cases, are totally unrelated to their principal job duties. These might include leadership, management, public speaking, writing, teaching, computer, artistic, and/or countless other skills. There are, in fact, a great many hidden talents in every employee.

ACTION STEP

Seek to identify the unique strengths and talents of each staff member," says Richard A. Green, DDS, MBA, director of Business Systems Development of the Pankey Institute. "Develop dynamic job descriptions and delegate tasks that amplify strengths and minimize weaknesses. People tend to grow more when they focus on success."[6]

176 Hard-learned lessons about performance reviews

Conducting performance reviews is often stressful for dentists and office managers as well as employees. *Avoiding* reviews, however, creates even more stress.

New employees should be evaluated shortly after they're hired, typically after 3 months. If a problem exists, it's least painful and least expensive for you and for them to discover it early. The new hire is a "go" or "no go." Don't waste time trying to rehabilitate someone who's a poor fit.

Don't discuss money in performance reviews. The issue on the table is the work, not the pay. Tell your employees before, during, and after performance reviews that you will be conducting compensation reviews later, but the issue today is improving performance.

The goal of the performance review should be improved performance in the future. Don't make the common mistake of putting undue focus on past performance.

"Sometimes, by interviewing employees, a doctor can discover the potential burnout or boredom that results from doing the same thing over and over," says author/consultant Cathy Jameson. "Often, you can defuse burnout by changing the job responsibility or switching people around. This switch may be temporary or you may discover that an employee blossoms in the new role, and you may encourage her or him to stay in the new position. Switching roles, exchanging responsibilities, or adding responsibilities can uncover tremendous potential within team members."[7]

"Performance reviews," says consultant Jeffrey J. Denning, "can help buttress your defense in the event you are sued by an employee (or more likely, a former employee). On the other hand, the absence of an evaluation or adequate review can sometimes be used against you with devastating results. Juries tend to come down hard on employers who don't appear to have given an employee a chance to improve. And the employee with no bad reviews who suddenly finds herself fired, is justified in being shocked—and you may be equally shocked when she sues for wrongful termination."[8]

177 Hard-learned lessons about firing employees

The most unpleasant and disliked task of practice management is the need to fire an employee. Most dentists detest the job.

The first thing to remember is there's no way to make a dismissal pleasant. You can only minimize the pain and hostility.

The following are some of the lessons that high-performance practitioners have learned about this task.

Lingering dismissals only prolong the agony for everyone.

Good employees resent those who do not carry their share of the work load.

Always fire someone face to face. The job can't be delegated anymore than it can be postponed.

Once you make the decision, "get 'em out quick." That's the overwhelming recommendation of the many personnel specialists I've asked about the timing of an employee's dismissal. The end of the day is preferred to avoid embarrassment for the employee. Mondays are preferred to Fridays so the person can go out on a Tuesday to look for other work rather than stew about it on the weekend.

Should you tell the employee reasons for your decision or gloss over them? Most personnel managers advocate an explanation somewhere between the two extremes. They advise giving the employee enough information to show your decision was not arbitrary, but not so much detail as to destroy the person's self-esteem in the process.

Stick to facts rather than feelings. Your opinions about a person's "attitude" or "personality" are debatable and will accomplish little except to inflict pain.

To avoid lawsuits claiming a wrongful dismissal, document everything as it occurs. When a problem is severe enough to require a warning, put it in writing, date it, and have the employee sign it. If it becomes necessary, this paper trail will provide a sound basis for a subsequent firing decision.

Adopt a low-key approach that the employee is just not right for your practice, in that job, at this time. Don't dwell on shortcomings. Simply express disappointment that things have not changed since the last performance review and that you have no alternative but to terminate employment. Acknowledge the person's capabilities and strong points. If appropriate, express regret that you don't have a job opening more suited to the person's qualifications, and let it go at that.

Tell other employees of your decision, indicating in simple terms the reasons for it and ask for their support until you find a replacement. Staff members may be more aware than you of the shortcomings of the former employee and actually applaud your decision.

FROM THE SUCCESS FILES

After a recent seminar, a dentist wrote me: "When I returned to my office, I fired my bookkeeper of 13 years. It was without doubt, the hardest, most painful thing I've ever done. It was also the best thing—

for my staff, my patients, and myself. It was hard to recognize the negative impact she had on the practice—until she left."

178 Exit interviews

Do you ever wonder about the level of morale among your employees or how they view their jobs, co-workers, and the day-to-day management of your practice? The answers could be helpful in improving productivity and practice growth.

Interviews with employees who voluntarily leave their jobs, called *exit interviews,* can often yield information that, for a variety of reasons, they're reluctant to tell you while still on the job.

TESTED TIP
To get honest feedback, assure departing employees of complete confidentiality and that what they say during the exit interview will not in any way be held against them (for example, if they ask for a reference).

SUGGESTED QUESTIONS
- "Are there any specific features of your new job that you feel were lacking in your job here?"
- "What did you think about the features of your job here such a salary, benefits, supervision, and office policies?"
- "What did you like best about your job here? What did you dislike about it?"
- "What suggestions do you have for us to make our office a better place to work?"
- "Were you satisfied or dissatisfied with the office environment? Are changes needed in the working space, lighting, heating, or air conditioning?"
- "How about the working conditions? Did you feel overworked? Underutilized?"
- "Were you under unusual stress?"
- "What were your real reasons for leaving our office? (Consider probing for the *critical factor* with follow-up questions such as

'What was the straw that broke the camel's back? When did you decide you wanted a different job?')"
- "Would you recommend our office as a good place to work?"
- All these questions may not fit each departing employee, so pick and choose as the situation warrants. During the questioning, it's best to be empathetic and non-judgmental. Comments such as "I wasn't aware of that; please go on" or "That's an interesting point; could you give me more details?" will encourage the employee to speak openly.

"The benefit to the practice," says consultant Linda Miles, "is to hopefully avoid losing staff for the same reason by identifying unfavorable traits in the employer or co-workers, unfair policies, or unmet expectations. The benefit to the doctor is discovering weaknesses he or she may not even know exist."[9]

REALITY CHECK

It's important to remember that departing employees are also "ambassadors" for your practice, whether you wish them to be or not. Even if they encountered several months of rough going before leaving, if the parting was amicable, they will be more inclined to speak favorably about the practice.

FROM THE SUCCESS FILES

The more I tried to educate my staff about promptness and perfection," admits ophthalmologist Dahlia Hirsch, MD, Bel Air, MD, "the worse the situation became. It wasn't because of the message, but how I delivered it. I often didn't appreciate what my employees did. I only noticed what they didn't or couldn't do. I was impatient. Sometimes I corrected them right in front of patients. My wake up call came one day when all four of my employees quit. We went to lunch, which became an exit interview of sorts and I asked them why they were quitting. I learned (painfully) that I was the reason. That lunch," she adds, "was the most valuable consultation I ever had. I realized that if I didn't change some patterns, I would have constant turnover."[10]

179 Hard-learned lessons about staff retention

It's far cheaper to retain good employees that it is to have to replace them.

Since launching their Web site, North Suburban Dental Associates in Skokie, IL, has found that *staff longevity* has proved to be an important element to the people who visit the site before showing up at the office. "We have found," says Barry Freydberg, DDS, "that staff longevity has been a major confidence builder in new patients we haven't met yet. We didn't know that this would have an influence on new patients but it has. Our credibility gets a boost based on staff longevity."[11]

"Good management is largely a matter of love. Or if you're uncomfortable with that word, call it caring, because proper management involves caring for people, not manipulating them." (James Autry)

Coddle your employees. Without them, you may not have a practice. If necessary, pay them before you pay yourself. Give them benefits you would not take for yourself. Spoil them and empower them in every way possible.

"Doctors should reward competence, encourage its development, and base all standards on excellence," advises the Blair/McGill Advisory. "That is why we encourage doctors to give individual raises based upon merit performance, not across-the-board cost of living increases that encourage mediocrity."[12]

"Don't give raises to marginal employees," says consultant Jeffrey J. Denning. "Raises never motivate workers to improve. To the contrary, a raise in pay signals the employer's satisfaction with status quo. Further, if an employee is terminated and sues, she has simply to point to the history of pay raises to show she was doing a good job. Judgment for the plaintiff."[8]

When staff members enjoy their work, their performance improves, leading to higher patient satisfaction and loyalty, which leads to more referrals and a reputation in the community as a "Provider of Choice."

People's on-the-job performance and productivity tend to improve when they know what's expected of them and receive periodic feedback about their work.

"It's not the people you fire who make your life miserable," says Harvey Mackay, "it's those you don't."[13]

Maybe you're a "glass half-empty" person and think your current employees are still captives in a sluggish economy. If so, here's a simple test. Do nothing, and see what happens.

Notes

1. How to Close the Revolving Door of Employee Turnover, *Blair/McGill Advisory,* June 2001, 4, 8.
2. Barbian J. Short Shelf Life. *Training,* June 2002, 50-52.
3. Skoch DA. Ask for Commitment, Not Loyalty. *Industry Week,* November 1994, 38.
4. Robbins SP. *The Truth About Managing People. And Nothing But The Truth.* Upper Saddle River, NJ: Financial Times Prentice-Hall, June 2003.
5. Weir JH. Performance Reviews: How to Make Them Great! *Dental Angle Online Magazine,* Fall 2001.
6. Green RA. A Great Place to Work! *Dental Economics,* July 2003, 56.
7. Jameson C. Review Time. *Dental Practice Report,* May 2001, 37-40.
8. How'm I Doin' Boss? *Uncommon Sense,* June 1997, 4.
9. Miles L. Measuring the Value of Exit Interviews. *Dental Practice Report,* October 2003, 17.
10. Hirsch D. How to Rediscover the Person in the Patient. *Review of Optometry,* July 1999.
11. Spaeth D. Winning Web Sites. *Dental Practice Report,* January/February 2002, 36-40.
12. How to Avoid the Seven Deadly Sins of Personnel Management, *Blair/McGill Advisory,* September 2003, 3.
13. Mackay H. *Swim With the Sharks.* New York: William Morrow & Co., 1988.

6. Having the goals and objectives of the practice spelled out so I know where we're headed
7. A written job description so I know what's expected of me
8. A good performance review so I know how I'm doing
9. Health insurance and other fringe benefits
10. The avoidance of criticism for doing an inadequate job
11. Maintenance of adequate living standards for my family
12. Being told by the doctor that I'm doing a good job
13. Getting along with coworkers
14. Participation in management activities
15. Involvement in decisions affecting my work
16. Feeling my job is important
17. Respect for me as a person and/or a professional at my job
18. Have more autonomy on the job
19. Have more job responsibilities
20. Interesting work
21. Opportunities to do work that is challenging
22. Chance for self-development and improvement

Others _____

REALITY CHECK

No two people have the same motivational needs or have them in the same order of importance. A single parent with two school-age children, for example, may have very different job-related needs than a person from a two wage–earner household with grown children.

Seminar audiences typically struggle with this Motivation Inventory, simply because it's difficult for them to know their employees' job-related needs unless they've discussed the subject with them.

ACTION STEP

To put employees' motivation in high gear (or keep it there) you must first identify their job-related needs and then make their jobs so satisfying that they will want, *really want*, to do their very best. Or as Bob Townsend, former CEO of Avis, has said, "Create the kind of environment that pays people to bring their brains to work."

182 Learn employees' job-related needs

There are several ways to learn about employees' needs.

Ideally, the initial job interview will uncover an applicant's job-related needs. The underlying purpose of many of the interview questions listed in Chapter 11 is to help you ascertain whether you have the right person for the right job in your office (e.g., "What about your last job did you like most? Least?").

Consider asking current employees similar questions to identify their job-related needs. In this case, put them in writing. Give them time to think about their answers, and perhaps discuss them with someone else. Explain also that if they'd like to do so, you'll schedule a one-on-one conference to discuss the results. Such questions might include the following:

- "What part of your job do you like best, and why?"
- "Are there additional things you would like to be doing?"
- "What, if anything, frustrates you about your job?"
- "What is there about your job (if anything) that you would like changed to help you get more of what you want from your work?"

"Ask your employees what is important to them and why they work for you when they have so many other opportunities," says Roger Herman, author of *Keeping Good People.* "Listen carefully to what they say, and then give them more of what they want. Then use those same factors to recruit, recognizing that the people you want will have similar desires to those who have chosen to be part of your team."[3]

The Motivation Inventory, although not intended for this purpose, can be used to identify employees' job-related needs.

Performance reviews (secret #174) are a more formal, in-depth way to learn employees' job-related needs.

The next step is to help employees get more of what they want from their work.

Here are some examples based on the Motivation Inventory.

183   Satisfactory working conditions

This item was number two in the Motivation Inventory.

Louis Harris did a survey of office workers regarding their "work environment." Not surprisingly, the factor considered most important was "good lighting." Number two was "comfortable seating," again, not surprising considering that back ailments affect 60-80% of the population and are the number two cause of absenteeism. (The number one cause is the common cold.)

What *is* surprising is how often employees complain about an "uncomfortable chair" in which they have to sit all day!

REALITY CHECK

Uncomfortable chairs contribute to more frequent stretch breaks, employee errors, and lower job satisfaction, *especially if employees complain about the problem and nothing is done.*

When a government department in New Jersey installed ergonomically correct workstations in their new offices, computer-related health complaints fell by 40% and doctor visits dropped by 25% in less than a year.

The study from Cornell University found that the 356 employees reported relief in all the places that hurt after a day of hunching over a keyboard: shoulders and neck, wrists and hands, and back. What made the difference? Chairs with adjustable armrests, backs, and seats; tilting keyboard holders; and mouse platforms. The workers also took regular breaks and stretched.[4]

Another related source of complaints: office and/or dental equipment that is out-of-date, frequently requires repair, and/or needs to be replaced.

The message to the employee in both the case of an uncomfortable chair and equipment that needs replacement is "You and your work are not important enough for me to remedy the situation."

REALITY CHECK

How friendly, understanding, or helpful are such disgruntled employees going to be when dealing with the patients in your practice?

184 The need for autonomy

This was number 18 in the Motivation Inventory.

"The ultimate form of recognition for many employees," says author/speaker Bob Nelson, PhD, "is to be given increased autonomy and authority to get their job done, whether it's the ability to spend or allocate resources, make decisions, or manage others. Greater autonomy and authority say in effect, 'I trust you to act in the best interests of the company, to do so independently and without approval of myself or others.'"

"Increased autonomy and authority," Nelson says, "should be awarded to employees as a form of recognition itself for past results they have achieved. Autonomy and authority are privileges, not rights, which should be granted to those who have most earned them, based on past performance, not based on tenure or authority."[5]

ACTION STEP

Let's use as an example the equipment described in the preceding secret that needs to be replaced. Empower the employee who uses the equipment on a daily basis to recommend (or buy outright) what's needed.

There are, of course, degrees of empowerment. Decide which is most appropriate based on the nature of the task and the abilities of the employee. For example, you can tell an employee any one of the following:

- Investigate the situation. Report back to me. I'll decide.
- Investigate. Make recommendations. I'll decide.
- Investigate. Decide. Let me have final approval.
- Take action. Let me know what you did.
- Whatever you do is OK with me.

REALITY CHECK

Empowerment to make such recommendations or decisions is extremely satisfying to people with a job-related need for autonomy and who seek more on-the-job responsibility and authority. In fact, many would consider it insulting *not* to be consulted in such matters.

A complaint I often hear from disgruntled employees is "I'm treated as if I don't have a brain in my head."

185 The need for interesting work

This was number 20 in the Motivation Inventory.

When asked, "What makes a job satisfying?" 30,000 readers of *Working Woman* magazine ranked "interesting and challenging work" number one.[6]

REALITY CHECK

It's been said that 75% of jobs can be learned in 3 years. For some people, doing the same thing every day is fine. For others, it results in boredom.

One of the best ways to make work more interesting is to give people with this need a chance to grow on the job. Tackle tasks that require what industrial psychologists call s-t-r-e-t-c-h. The principle involved is as follows: *The competence of most people is increased when they are given a challenge.* It's the same principle as playing a sport with someone who's a *little* better at it than you. The sport could be ping-pong, dancing, or Scrabble. Playing with such a partner or opponent is motivational—it makes you perform better. That's s-t-r-e-t-c-h. And because you play better, you also have a *sense of achievement.*

ACTION STEPS

The following are among the ways to make a job more interesting:

* *Cross-training.* Gives employees an opportunity to try different jobs in the office. Cross-training provides a change-of-pace and avoids burn out. It helps everyone better understand the demands of each other's jobs, and promotes teamwork.

FROM THE SUCCESS FILES

"We make a huge investment in cross-training our staff on everything in our office," say Roy Hammond, DDS, and Chris Hammond, DMD, Provo, UT. "Everyone has to know all the procedures when there is an illness or other events occur."[7]

* *Continuing education programs.* These enable employees to learn new clinical, laboratory, and office-related skills.

• *Job enrichment*. This involves additional responsibilities such as developing the practice Web site, writing a patient newsletter, and doing public relations for the practice.

HARD-LEARNED LESSON

It's achievement that leads to motivation, not the other way around. You see it in the "high fives" that athletes trade after scoring a touchdown or hitting a homerun. You see it in the expression of someone on a diet who discovers after weeks of self-discipline that he's lost 5 pounds.

The point is, if you want to motivate employees, don't lecture them. Don't threaten them with dismissal if they don't improve. Instead, provide *s-t-r-e-t-c-h* and opportunities for growth.

ACTION STEP

Ask employees what specific knowledge and skills they'd like to learn. Then design a program that incorporates the needs of individuals as well as the practice itself.

---

186 The desire for on-the-job training

Staff training is most appealing to people who have such job-related needs as the following:

Number 19, more job responsibilities; number 20, interesting work; number 21, opportunities to do work that is challenging; and number 22, the chance for self-development and improvement. For many, it is the key to job satisfaction.

Among the topics you might consider for in-service training: Occupational Safety and Health Administration (OSHA) and Health Insurance Portability and Accountability Act (HIPAA) review, clinical assisting, office computers/practice management software systems, communication with patients, CPR and other patient emergency procedures, dental insurance filing and coding, and explaining financial policies to patients.

"All team members need to know the basics of insurance," says consultant Kathy Mohr, "so they can answer some of those 'will my insurance cover this' questions."[8]

ACTION STEP

"Encourage your employees to take full advantage of CE offerings," advises the American Dental Association catalog. "A practice resource center where employees can check out manuals, books, multimedia programs, and other products is another great way to allow employees access to training materials."[9]

FROM THE SUCCESS FILES

"In our offices, we train, train, and retrain," says Hal Ornstein, DPM, Howell, NJ. "With the dynamic nature of medicine and the insurance industry, our staff is trained in several fashions to stay on top. At first, we were afraid of the extra cost associated with training a new employee. We've since learned that investing in training new employees delivers an awesome return."[10]

187 Hard-learned lessons about training

"Nobody should perform the same task all the time," says author/speaker Marvin H. Berman, DDS, Chicago, IL. "Beware the employee who says, 'I'm the only one who knows how to do that.'"[11]

"As dentistry's advance toward new technology continues," says Dennis Spaeth, editor of *Dental Practice Report*, "staff training promises to play an increasingly critical role in dental practice—particularly with a growing number of practice management software applications that work in concert with such equipment as intraoral cameras and digital radiography."[12]

An article in *Fortune* titled "Managing for the Slowdown" stresses the importance of quality employees. "We hope it's no longer necessary to argue that this is increasingly your company's only source of competitive advantage . . . Getting the best people and making them better is in the DNA of the most successful companies."[13]

Don't send your ducks to eagle school. Training someone who wishes only for a paycheck is as pointless and self-defeating as placing someone with a desire for professional growth in a repetitive, dead-end job.

Surprisingly, some dentists say they can't afford to train because of the expense and because better-trained, more highly skilled employees may decide to leave for better opportunities. That's true. But training new employees and having them leave is not nearly as bad as *not* training them and having them stay.

188 The need for appreciation

This was number 12 in the Motivation Inventory.

In an Internet survey conducted by best-selling author Bob Nelson, PhD, 87.9% of 762 respondents ranked "being personally thanked for doing good work" as either "extremely important" or "very important." Of the respondents, 60.8% did the same for "being praised for good work in front of others."[14]

Finding something nice to say about others may seem trivial, but it satisfies a universal hunger. Unfortunately, people who feel appreciation often fail to express it. They become inhibited, forgetful, and busy with other day-to-day priorities.

Many dental staff members I've interviewed feel most thwarted and frustrated about their work because of a lack of appreciation. Included are those who do above-average work, but receive no special recognition or appreciation. Many have said, "The only time I get any feedback about my work is when I make a mistake." They believe their efforts to do a good job are never even *noticed*, let alone appreciated.

Some dentists mistakenly assume their employees' need for appreciation can be *internally* met ("She knows she does a good job"). Even if that were true, a verbal pat on the back or a written note of thanks for a "job well done" provides the kind of psychological satisfaction for which there is absolutely no substitute.

When President Reagan wrote "Very Good" on the draft of a speech prepared by speech writer Peggy Noonan, she cut the words out, taped them to her blouse, and wore them all day.

ACTION STEP
Systematically start to thank your staff members when they do good work, whether it's one-on-one in person, in the hallway, at a staff

meeting, on voicemail, in a written thank-you note, on e-mail, or at the end of each day at work.

I guarantee it'll make their day, and by expressing appreciation, you may start a chain reaction. Praise begets praise. People will like you more for saying kind things, and you'll feel good for having said them.

REALITY CHECK

How often do you give out praise? More to the point, how often have you failed to do so in situations in which praise was truly deserved?

189 Hard-learned lessons about appreciation

Appreciation results in short-term motivation.

Achievement leads to long-term motivation.

One clue to a job applicant's need for appreciation is his or her answer to the question: "In your last job, did you receive the recognition and appreciation, you felt you deserved?"

People differ in what they want to be applauded and appreciated for, says Marc Albin, CEO of a high-tech staffing consulting company in Sunnyvale, CA, depending on what personal qualities and talents they're most proud of. "My experience in managing people is they're all different," he says. "Some want to be recognized for the quality of their work, some for the quantity of their work. Some people want to be recognized for their cheerful attitude and their ability to spread their cheerful attitude. Some like to be recognized individually; others want to be recognized in groups. No one has ever said, 'Just recognize me for anything I do well.'" To identify which parts of individual employees' egos need scratching, Albin takes an unconventional approach: he asks them.[15]

"Recognize, reinforce, and praise your employees for work well done and for accomplishments," says consultant/speaker Cathy Jameson, PhD. "Positive reinforcement solidifies excellent behavior or excellent work. Positive reinforcement far outshines negative reinforcement in getting desired results. Whether it comes in the form of a formal recognition, such as a bonus check, or as informal recognition, such as a compliment, you will find that this reinforcement may be the most important thing you can do for employee satisfaction."[16]

190 The need to have a say in decisions affecting one's work

This was number 15 in the Motivation Inventory.

REALITY CHECK

The motivation to accomplish results tends to increase as people are given an opportunity to participate in the decisions affecting those results.

Sharing decision-making power demonstrates respect for employees and their expertise and increases the likelihood of better decisions. It also helps your employees develop a sense of ownership of their jobs, which, in turn, makes their work more motivating and satisfying.

Equally important: When employees feel they have some say in the decisions that vitally affect their work, they're more highly motivated to perform with distinction than if they feel they're merely being told what to do.

ACTION STEP

"Ask for your team members' opinions on materials, delivery systems, and equipment selection," says Lori Trost, DMD, Editor of *Woman Dentist Journal*. "After all, they are the ones who will be using them. Their input is invaluable."[17]

HARD-LEARNED LESSON

"At Mary Kay Cosmetics," said Mary Kay Ash, "we want our people's ideas. We encourage them and openly solicit them. Their participation is vital to our growth and health. The more that people are permitted to participate in a new project, the more they'll support it. Conversely, the more they are excluded, the more they will resist it."[18]

191 Hard-learned lessons about motivation

The question isn't "How do I get my employees to do what I want them to do?" Rather, it's "How do I get my employees *to want to do* what I want them to do?"

Trying to motivate others without understanding their job-related motivational needs is like trying to start a stalled car by kicking it.

"Money attracts and retains people," says consultant Jon R. Katzenbach, "better than it motivates them to excel."[19]

Prove the significance of your employees. Make sure everyone on your staff feels famous for something. You want them to always have a reason to come to work.

Whenever possible, implement changes in office policies and procedures by *consensus*. People tend to be more supportive of decisions in which they have some input. *And*, they're more interested in seeing a successful outcome than they are of decisions made by others and passed along to them to implement.

"A vital factor in morale," said David Ogilvy, who built one of the largest advertising agencies in the world, "is the posture of the boss. If he or she is miserable, it will filter down through the ranks, and make the whole office miserable. You must always be contagiously cheerful."[20]

"People who work in a fulfilling work environment," says Tom Chappell, co-founder and president of personal-care product manufacturer Tom's of Maine, "where they feel both valued and respected, are more productive and loyal."[21]

Almost without exception, good work that goes unnoticed and unappreciated tends to deteriorate.

Some people would rather have *praise* than a *raise*.

Money motivates people, but only up to a point.

REALITY CHECK

If you gave every employee a $1000 raise starting tomorrow, how much harder would they work, and for how long?

192 Assess the motivational climate in your practice

What are the core elements needed to attract and retain top-notch employees in the current marketplace, and does your practice have them?

In their book, *First Break All the Rules,* Marcus Buckingham and Curt Coffman discuss research on these topics conducted by the Gallup Organization. The massive, in-depth study correlated performance data from more than 2500 business units and opinion data from over 105,000 employees. ("The definition of a business unit varied by industry: for banking, it was the branch; for hospitality, it was the restaurant or hotel; for manufacturing, it was the factory; and so on.")

After extensive analysis (including a combination of focus groups, factor analysis, regression analysis, concurrent validity studies, and follow-up interviews) the following 12 questions were used to measure what the authors call the *"strength of a workplace."* Although these questions don't capture everything you want to know about a workplace, they do measure the core elements needed to "attract, focus, and keep the most talented employees."

How would your employees answer these questions on a 1-5 scale, in which "1" equals strongly disagree and "5" equals strongly agree?

1. "Do I know what is expected of me?"
2. "Do I have the materials and equipment I need to do my work right?"
3. "At work, do I have the opportunity to do what I do best every day?"
4. "In the last 7 days, have I received recognition or praise for good work?"
5. "Does my supervisor, or someone at work, seem to care about me as a person?"
6. "Is there someone at work who encourages my development?"
7. "At work, do my opinions seem to count?"
8. "Does the mission/purpose of my company make me feel like my work is important?"
9. "Are my co-workers committed to doing quality work?"
10. "Do I have a best friend at work?"

11. "In the last 6 months, have I talked with someone about my progress?"
12. "At work, have I had opportunities to learn and grow?"

What the authors found was that "those employees who responded more positively to the twelve questions also worked in business units with higher levels of productivity, profit, retention, and customer satisfaction. This demonstrated for the first time the link between employee opinion and business unit performance, across many different companies."

You may be wondering why no questions deal with pay, benefits, or advancement. "There were initially," say the authors, "but they disappeared during the analysis. This doesn't mean they're unimportant. It simply means they are equally important to every employee, good, bad, or mediocre. Yes, if you are paying 20 percent below the market average, you may have difficulty attracting people. But bringing your pay and benefit package up to market levels, while a sensible first step, will not take you very far. These kinds of issues are like tickets to the ballpark—they can get you into the game, but they can't help you win."[22]

ACTION STEP

By *guessing* how your employees would answer these questions (or, if you have the courage, actually *learning* first-hand) you can evaluate the motivational climate in your practice and perhaps identify what, if anything, is needed to improve it.

Notes

1. Bell CR, Zemke R. *Managing Knock Your Socks Off Service.* AMACOM, 1992, 203.
2. Wilbur J, Tse D. It Starts With the Right People. *Dental Economics,* June 2003.
3. How to Build IT Loyalty. *Workforce,* July 2001, 53.
4. Rudakewych M, Valent-Weitz L, Hedge A. Effects of an Ergonomic Intervention on Musculoskeletal Discomfort Among Office Workers, Proceedings of the Human Factors and Ergonomics Society 45th Annual Meeting, Vol. 1, 791-795.
5. maillist@nelson-motivation.com, September 4, 2002.
6. Ciabattari J. The Biggest Mistake Top Managers Make. *Working Woman,* October 1996, 47-55.
7. Henry K. Office Spotlight. *Dental Equipment & Materials,* January/February 2004, 8-10.
8. Mohr K. Collection—A Team Effort. *Insurance Solutions,* July/August 2000, 9.

9. ADA 2004 Annual Catalog, www.adacatalog.com, accessed 9/4/04.
10. Guiliana JV, Vance CE, Schiraldi-Deck FG, et al. Roundtable: Staff Management. *Podiatry Management,* January 2001, 93-106.
11. Berman MH. Tips from a Fellow Traveler, Part 1. *Dental Economics,* February 2000.
12. Spaeth D. Staff Training for the High-Tech Office. *Dental Practice Report,* May 2003.
13. Charan R, Colvin G. Managing for the Slowdown. *Fortune,* February 2001.
14. Nelson B. *What Do Employees Want? Employee Recognition Practices Inventory,* www.nelson-motivation.com.
15. Buchanan L. Managing One-to-One. *Inc. Magazine,* October 2001, 83-89.
16. Jameson C. Six Strategies for Keeping Talented Team Members. *Dental Practice Report,* May 2001, 39.
17. Trost L. Building Your Dream Team. *Woman Dentist Journal,* March/April 2003, 62-66.
18. Krauss P. *The Book of Management Wisdom: Classic Writings by Legendary Managers.* New York: John Wiley & Sons, Inc., 2000.
19. Katzenbach JR. *Why Pride Matters More Than Money.* New York, Crown Business, 2003.
20. Ogilvy D. *Blood, Brains & Beer,* New York: Atheneum, 1978.
21. Finnigan A. Benefits Under Fire. *Working Woman,* July/August 2001, 54, 56, 58, 78.
22. Buckingham M, Coffman C. *First, Break All the Rules.* New York: Simon & Schuster, 2004.

15

Action Steps to Ignite Practice Growth

The day before conducting a seminar in Vancouver, British Columbia, Canada, for the Continuing Legal Education Society of British Columbia, I met with a prominent attorney in Vancouver. He told me how crowded and competitive the law profession had become in his province. There were fewer clients because of mergers, acquisitions, and in-house counsels. There was an increase in non-lawyers who now offer services that were once the province of lawyers. "We used to walk through the forest," he said, "and the nuts would just fall out of the trees. That's not happening today."

The underlying reasons, of course, are different, but the forest analogy is also true for dentistry.

REALITY CHECK
What you've done to get your practice where it is today is no longer adequate to keep it there.

Here are some final action steps to put you "on target" for a high-performance dental practice.

193 Set goals

"Set goals," says pedodontist James B. Jackson, Pleasant, SC. "Don't just let things happen. Make them happen. Establish both short- and long-term goals."[1]

Goal setting helps you discover what you really want to accomplish in life, both personally and professionally. It forces you to make commitments and reduces unnecessary conflict over what to do. Writing goals down on a sheet of paper goes a step further. It makes them more specific and concrete. Once goals have a visible identity, they can be scrutinized more closely: analyzed, refined, and pondered. When conditions or values change, they can be updated, altered, or perhaps abandoned.

Substantial evidence exists that goals are more achievable if they are broken down into their most manageable parts. For example, for most of his NBA career, Michael Jordan kept his scoring average at 32 points per game. He retired in 1999 with an NBA record of a 31.5-point career average. It didn't matter who his teammates were, what defense they were running, what injuries he was nursing, or who was guarding him. Michael Jordan would get his 32 points.

When reporters asked him how he consistently maintained that average for more than a decade, Jordan said, "I simplified it a few years ago. 32 points per game is really just 8 points a quarter. I figure I can get that in some kind of way during the course of a game."

ACTION STEP

Make a detailed list of the practice goals that are most meaningful to you. These can include, says consultant James R. Pride, DDS, Novato, CA, such goals as "production per hour, collection percentage, accounts receivable over 60 and 90 days, case acceptance rate, allowable amount of managed care or write-offs, number of cancellations or no-shows, and on-time starts and finishes."[2] Then break them down into manageable, bite-sized, mini-goals.

Goals need to be specific, measurable, and attainable objectives that everyone in the office should be working toward daily, said seminar speaker Walter Hailey. "In fact, the more clear-cut you make the goals of your practice," he added, "the more dramatically you reduce the chance of confusion, conflict, and frustration among your team. Post the goals in a place where all team members can see them every day. Make it clear where the practice is headed."[3]

FROM THE SUCCESS FILES

"We worked on a changeover from a standard general practice to a cosmetic dentistry general practice by setting goals every six months," says Stephen D. Poss, DDS, Smyrna, TN. "Once those goals were achieved, we re-evaluated our status and set new goals for the next six months. One of the first goals entailed eliminating those procedures I did not wish to continue such as full and partial dentures, extractions, endodontics, and pediatric dentistry. We eliminated amalgam and converted to a metal-free practice. Our goals focused on marketing issues, staff and patient education, and equipment purchases."[4]

REALITY CHECK

"I think setting goals is important," says Lynn Carlisle, DDS, Fort Collins, CO. "It is something I think should be done yearly in your personal and professional life. Will you reach all of your goals? I don't think so. If you don't reach a goal, look at it and see if corrections would lead to achieving the goal. Make the corrections without invalidating yourself."

"If it isn't achievable, let it go . . . Move on to something else. Sometimes the magic works and sometimes it doesn't."

"See what life brings you."[5]

194 Soar with your strengths

"Find out what you do well—and do more of it. Find out what you don't do well—and stop doing it." That recommendation comes from the book, *Soar With Your Strengths*, by Donald O. Clifton, PhD, and Paula Nelson.

Strengths, the authors say, are things that you do well and learn easily, that produce a high degree of satisfaction and pride, and that generate psychological and/or financial rewards. Weaknesses are those things you don't do well and at which you don't significantly improve even after repeated tries. They intrude on your productivity and self-esteem and cause undue stress. No matter how dedicated you may be to improving yourself, the authors say, you'll never transform weaknesses into strengths.

ACTION STEP

The goal is to concentrate on your strengths and manage your weaknesses. One technique: Delegate tasks you don't do well or enjoy to those whose strengths lie in these areas. Then use your time for more constructive pursuits.

"I struggled for a while with the hiring, management, and occasional firing of employees in our office," an Illinois dentist admitted, "but I wasn't good at it—and I didn't like the job. One of my partners, much better suited for these matters, took over—and everyone's happier, employees included."

Some of the happiest dentists I know are those who have concentrated their efforts on what they do well and enjoy doing.

"Most dentists tell me they want to focus their practice on crown and bridge and restorative dentistry," writes Howard Farran, DDS, MBA, MAGD, Publisher of *Dentaltown Magazine*. "It's soooo simple," it continues. "You just have to master the 'Team Approach.' You have to get completely connected to all those weird dentists around the corner from you who enjoy molar endo, removing impacted wisdom teeth, doing quadrant gum surgeries, listening to screaming children with baby bottle tooth decay, and dealing with moms during ortho."[6]

FROM THE SUCCESS FILES

"I constantly feel energized about what I do now that I have focused my practice on adhesive dentistry," says Christopher Pescatore, DMD, Danville, CA. "I no longer have to run from room to room to see patients. I can spend more time with each patient and build valuable relationships, something I could never do in a larger practice setting. A typical day for me is seeing anywhere from one to six patients, depending on the procedures that I'm performing. I usually work a four-day week from 8:30 a.m. to 4:45 p.m., with a one-hour lunch break."[7]

HARD-LEARNED LESSON

Identifying weaknesses and emphasizing strengths in yourself and others is one of the most valuable and liberating discoveries you can make. It's also the surest route to achieving a high-performance dental practice.

195 Be good on the basics

"The most important thing," says J.W. Marriott, founder of the Marriott Corporation, "is to serve the hot food hot and the cold food cold."

He's talking of course, about the importance of *basics,* and it's as true about dental service as it is about food service. You may have sunk a fortune into the design of your office, and have the newest and best equipment on the market, but if you and your staff don't deliver on what patients consider the *basics* of good service, you've missed the boat. Big time.

What are the basics? They're the fundamental things that decide whether or not patients pay their bills cheerfully and promptly, remain loyal to your practice, and refer others to you.

Marriott identified its basics by analyzing the results of a comprehensive guest survey. They learned that guests' intent to return rests on five critical factors: everything is clean and works, check-in is hassle free, staff is friendly and helpful, problems are resolved quickly, and breakfast is served on time.

When Marriott fails to deliver on these basic expectations, guests have an unsatisfactory stay at a Marriott hotel. And no amount of mints on the pillow will bring back a guest who had to wait 30 minutes to check in, whose bathroom was dirty, and whose breakfast was overcooked and late in coming.

FROM THE SUCCESS FILES

"Practicing near the campus of Brigham Young University and several technology-oriented corporations," say Chris Hammond, DDS, and Roy Hammond, DMD, Provo, UT, "we know that high-tech is high on the priority list of many of our patients."

"Provo is a college town, but it is also a high-tech town," they add. "Our patients know, and we know, that the more time you can use technology in the dental office, the more time we will have to spend with the patients. If you want high-tech employees to choose your practice, you have to have a high-tech office."[8]

ACTION STEPS

Decide with your staff what basic services matter most to your patients. Use the following statement and fill in the blanks: "Nothing else matters if we don't _____ or aren't _____."

This is one of the exercises I have seminar audiences do. Answers have included: be available for emergencies, on time for appointments, have a high-tech office, have a meticulously clean office, answer patients' questions.

Be good on the basics and patients will tolerate almost anything else. Screw up on the basics and nothing else matters. Patients won't return. Period.

---

196 Develop a niche practice

"While there are a few 'decathlon dentists' who do everything well," says Tom Trinkner, DDS, Columbia, SC, "most dentists narrow their practices somewhat."[9]

At one time, the *mass market* was every dentist's target population. The trend today, however, is to pursue a "niche marketing" strategy. This strategy means targeting a specific population of patients, identifying their needs, and then addressing those needs more competently than anyone else.

Also, by focusing on a specific segment of the population, you're more likely to know what those patients want and provide them with a higher level of satisfaction than you are trying to be all things to all people.

FROM THE SUCCESS FILES

Because of a growing, affluent Japanese community in Westchester County, NY, Richard M. Crain, DMD, Larchmont, NY, hired a Japanese dental assistant and, with her help, began learning some basic phrases. He also installed a phone line with an answering message in Japanese and had his dental forms translated into Japanese. The plan worked. At last count, he has treated more than 500 Japanese patients.[10]

"Frank Hodges, DDS, Santa Rosa, CA, knew that in a community of some 200 dentists, he would have to differentiate his practice," writes consultant/speaker Deborah Walton. "After reviewing the market needs, he decided to specialize in children's services—effectively reducing his competition from 200 to 5. But rather than limit his market to just children, he redesigned his offices to also serve young adults. With the help of a consultant, out went the toys and decorations that gave the office a child-like appearance and in came colorful silk banners, photographs of animals, individual headsets and music libraries for teens, and more. He also joined the local school board and the board of the area Girl Scout council."[11]

"According to the ADA and NIH," says Jack Bynes, DMD, Coventry, CT, "there are 40 million Americans who avoid dentistry because of their fear. Not only is it a huge market, but it's one that's comprised of a population needing a tremendous amount of periodontal, endodontic, and restorative dentistry as opposed to elective dentistry."

Developing a practice centered on anxious and phobic patients, Dr. Bynes says, has numerous advantages. "You will avoid the hazards of managed care and insurance companies because phobic patients are willing to pay more out of pocket to be treated the way they should be treated—with kindness, patience and compassion. Eventually, such patients will become candidates for elective dentistry as their fears subside and their self-images improve. Another advantage is the unusually high number of referrals these patients generate."[12]

HARD-LEARNED LESSON
You've got to choose your strategy carefully. There's no point rowing harder if you're rowing in the wrong direction.

197 Combine your interests

The office of Peter Silver, DDS, New York, NY, caters to jazz musicians, many of whom are celebrities. The key to his success? He understands their concerns about embouchure (the manner in which the mouth and lips are applied to the mouthpiece of their instruments) because Dr. Silver himself is a highly accomplished trumpet player. He also leads a 17-piece big band and brass quintet during his off-hours.

Playing wind and brass instruments, Dr. Silver explained, is a complex neuromuscular task: groups of muscles function together to produce the necessary stream of air. "Someone might have an anterior tooth restoration replaced by another dentist," he says, "and all of a sudden he or she has trouble playing and doesn't understand why. And there's no training for this in dental school. If a restoration or a veneer is a millimeter too far forward, that could cause a trumpet player to start losing his or her high register."

"Most dentists," Dr. Silver adds, "think about how they can improve a person's smile or occlusion, but in the process, the patient can lose his or her ability to play. I have players bring their instruments to the office, sit in the chair, and play a little bit beforehand. After we make an adjustment, they play again and see how it feels. I can hear differences in their tone. The sound may center more when the lip has room to vibrate properly."

People who like jazz love Dr. Silver's office where jazz is played non-stop throughout the day and the walls are lined with photos from prominent jazz musicians with personalized messages thanking Dr. Silver for saving their "chops."

"I'm passionate about two things," Dr. Silver told me, "dentistry and jazz. This type of practice is a great way to combine the two of them."

198 Reposition your practice

Sometimes niche markets don't work out. The reasons vary.

During a seminar I conducted in Michigan, a dentist seemed skeptical that he could upgrade his practice and his patient's thinking about quality dentistry.

"I practice in a blue collar community," he said. "There are 25,000 people employed in automobile plants—at which there are frequent layoffs. It's a very price-conscious community. These ideas won't work here."

"How many middle- and top-management people work at those automobile plants?" I asked.

"A couple of thousand," he guessed

"Who has these as patients?" I asked the audience.

There was a long pause. Then, from the back of the room, the hand of another dentist went up.

"I do," he said.

The point seemed to have been made and I continued the lecture. Several years later I learned that particular exchange set the wheels in motion for a revitalized (and repositioned) practice for that same dentist who said, "It won't work here."

FROM THE SUCCESS FILES

"My philosophy," says Corky Willhite, DDS, Metairie, LA, "has always been to do the best dentistry possible. Because I have to spend more time with patients to accomplish that, my fees have always been high for my area. Throughout time, my practice has gradually gained patients who place a high value on their teeth and smile. They appreciate that the type of care I provide costs more because it takes more time and skill. And although most of my patients have to budget their finances, they prioritize their dental care above other purchases, such as vacations or new cars. These patients are very different from most of my early patients who seemed more interested in how much insurance would cover than in what was best for them."[13]

199 Decide what you want to be famous for

Midwest Express Airlines, for example, chooses to be famous for "The best care in the air," its signature statement in all its advertising, and they walk their talk. Coach passengers are treated as though they're flying first class. There are no middle seats. The seats are larger than average, leather, and comfortable. Full meals are served on china along with complimentary wine or champagne and chocolate chip cookies— freshly baked on board. And the flight attendants are invariably friendly. In a commodity-like industry, Midwest Express is a non-commodity player with a very loyal following.

The positioning strategy of Federal Express is based on a simple promise: "When it absolutely, positively has to be there overnight."

These lofty aspirations set the stage. They simplify the task of day-to-day operation, and make it easier for everyone to stay focused and, as the politicians say, "on message."

200 Give people something to talk about

"When more than 500 of your patients work at Microsoft, your office has to be high-tech," writes Kevin Henry, editor of *Dental Equipment & Materials.* "But for those 500+ patients to refer their friends and coworkers to your practice, your office better be high-touch as well."

This is the line that Kent Smith, DDS, and Jeff Roy, DDS, walk every day at 21st Century Dental in Irving, Texas.

"When part of your patient base works at Microsoft, and part of your patient base works at Verizon, those patients are going to know what high-tech options are out there for dentists," says Dr. Smith. "Having a computer chairside and digital radiography in the office is a must."

"A reception area, complete with beverage center and a 42-inch plasma monitor for cable TV, DVDs, or videos, is the focal point of the front office. Also included in the front room are a saltwater coral reef aquarium and a commissioned fresco. Glass blocks line the office and warm cookies and fresh flowers give 21st Century Dental a wonderful smell."

"I want these people to walk in our office and say 'Wow,'" says Dr. Smith. "I want them to think they have never been to a dental office like this. A lot of our patients are in their 20s or 30s and work around here. They don't come to see us and go home. They go back to work. I want them to go back to work talking about us and our office."[14]

201 Start today

Schedule a "no-holds-barred" staff meeting to brainstorm some of the questions posed in this book such as:

- What are the greatest strengths of the practice?
- What are the compliments most frequently heard about the practice?
- Why has the practice been successful?
- Do we need, at this time, to have different priorities? Develop new strengths?

- What accounts for patient loyalty?
- What is our competitive advantage?
- How can we develop an "emotional connection" with patients?
- What are the core values of our practice?
- What is the "personality" of our practice?
- What do we want to be famous for?
- What are the 'basics" of serving our patients?
- What are the weaknesses of the practice?
- What should we be doing that we're not doing?
- How can we be easier to do business with? (E.T.D.B.W.)
- What opportunities for improved profitability and practice growth make the most sense for us in the coming year?
- What is the perceived value of treatment in our office compared to the fees charged?
- What threats to practice growth do we face in the year ahead?
- What will our Action Plan be for the year ahead?

When we divide seminar audiences into small discussion groups (by practice) for this exercise, the excitement builds. Before long, everyone is animated and participating. Sparks fly. One idea acts as a springboard for others, and creative thinking is stimulated. Lists are started of the changes needed, projects to start, goals to achieve, and timetables for completion. The high-performance practice is set in motion.

Go for it!

Notes

1. Jackson JB. Six Paths to Success. *The Press Report.*
2. Pride JR. Regression to the Mean. *Dental Economics,* November 2000, 98-103.
3. Hailey W. Your New Year's Resolution List. *Dental Persuasion,* January/February 1997, Vol. 5, Issue 1.
4. Poss SD. How to Profit from Endodontics. *Dental Economics,* February 1999.
5. Carlisle L. Should You Set Yearly Goals for Your Dental Practice and Life? www.SpiritofCaring.com, accessed 9/4/04.
6. Farran H. Take Your Study Club to the Next Level. *Dentaltown,* May 2004, 6, 8.
7. Pescatore C. The Wonderful World of Adhesive Dentistry. *Dental Economics,* July 2003, 46-50.
8. Henry K. Office Spotlight. *Dental Equipment & Materials,* January/February 2004, 8-10.
9. Allen J. Shortening the Learning Curve. *AACD Journal,* Winter 1997, 49-55.
10. Mohn T. All Aboard the Foreign Language Express. *The New York Times,* October 11, 2000.

11. Walton D. Branding Your Practice. *Dental Practice & Finance,* November/December 1997, 25-26.
12. Bynes J. Shaping Your Practice. *Dental Economics,* March 2004, 139-141.
13. Bonner P. Integrating Cosmetic Dentistry into the General Dental Practice. *Dentistry Today,* April 1999, 45.
14. Henry K. Office Spotlight: Combining High-Tech With High-Touch. *Dental Equipment & Materials,* September 2000.

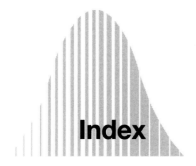

Index